The Institute of Biology's
Studies in Biology no. 7

# Guts
## The Form and Function
## of the Digestive System

## Second Edition

## John Morton
D.Sc.(Lond)

Professor of Zoology, University of Auckland, New Zealand

Edward Arnold

*First published 1967*
by Edward Arnold (Publishers) Limited,
41 Bedford Square, London WC1B 3DQ
*Second edition 1979*

**British Library Cataloguing in Publication Data**

Morton, John, b. 1923
    Guts. – 2nd ed. – (Institute of Biology. Studies
    in biology; no. 7   ISSN 0537–9024).
    1.   Intestines
    I.   Title.   II.   Series.
    591.1'3'2      QL863

ISBN 0–7131–2735–X

Printed and bound in Great Britain at
The Camelot Press Ltd, Southampton

# General Preface to the Series

Because it is no longer possible for one textbook to cover the whole field of biology while remaining sufficiently up to date the Institute of Biology has sponsored this series so that teachers and students can learn about significant developments. The enthusiastic acceptance of 'Studies in Biology' shows that the books are providing authoritative views of biological topics.

The features of the series include the attention given to methods, the selected list of books for further reading and, wherever possible, suggestions for practical work.

Readers' comments will be welcomed by the Education Officer of the Institute.

1979

Institute of Biology
41 Queen's Gate
London SW7 5HU

# Preface to the Second Edition

Since the first edition in 1967 the study of the gut has advanced on many fronts. These advances were made possible by new physiological methods, such as radio-isotope biology and partition chromatography, and perhaps most of all by the continued use of the electron microscope, an instrument that has given new life and direction to histology. This book has been revised to include a balanced view of what is new, but its old basis has been retained.

One of the merits of the gut system for study is that it is the first and most obtrusive of the great systems a student finds in dissection, and it is a system whose complexity is easy to study. The gut can be studied at a variety of levels from the ecological to the biochemical, and the basic theme of this book is the diversity of gut function at all these levels. Diversity is one of the great themes of biology, and a study of the gut reveals the lavish diversity and design for particular function that is characteristic of all living organisms.

Auckland, 1978

J. E. M.

# Contents

# 1 Introduction: Function and Diversity

## 1.1 Intracellular digestion

In common with all living organisms animals need a supply of energy. This energy comes from food which must be ingested, taken into the animal, and then prepared for use by the process of digestion. Both ingestion and digestion can occur without a gut. At its simplest ingestion consists of the movement of molecules across a cell or body wall, as happens in protozoans in a culture of dissolved organic material and in some internal parasites. Ingestion can also occur at the cellular level by the process of endocytosis. Pinocytosis (cell drinking) is one kind of endocytosis where droplets of dissolved material are engulfed into a closed vesicle by overarching of the cell membrane, or the pinching off of droplets from tubular invaginations. Within this vesicle cell-wall permeability is lowered and water and solutes diffuse freely into the surrounding cytoplasm. Phagocytosis (cell eating), the other kind of endocytosis, involves the engulfment of particles larger than molecules.

Digestion also varies from one animal to another. In some animals digestion is wholly intracellular; the food passes directly into the cell cytoplasm by phagocytosis and is attacked in food vacuoles by digestive enzymes. More commonly, however, extracellular digestion occurs, although the final stages of digestion may remain intracellular.

The process of intracellular digestion can be observed in the food vacuoles of protozoans. The formation of ingestion vacuoles (phago-somes) in *Amoeba* can readily be followed if Indian ink is added to the food. A certain amount of water is taken in with the food and the vacuoles have at first smooth contours. A minute or so later the vacuoles become invested by granules that stain intensely for acid phosphatase, which is a characteristic of lysosomes. As the ingestion vacuole reduces in size due to loss of water, the lysosomes pour their enzymes into the vacuole which then becomes a digestion vacuole. The amorphous products of digestion gather near the vacuole membrane, which now becomes drawn out into finger-like processes greatly increasing the interface with the cytoplasm, and then move out by 'micro-pinocytosis'. At this stage acid phosphatase cannot be detected and the vacuole becomes simply an egestion vacuole discharging its contents from the cell by exocytosis (Fig. 1–1a).

It is believed that enzymes enclosed in the membranous organelles called lysosomes are present in all cells. Lysosomes are generally identified by the reaction for acid phosphatase, although their enzyme complement includes various carbohydrases (breaking down glycogen and mucopolysaccharides); a range of peptidases (amino-, exo- and

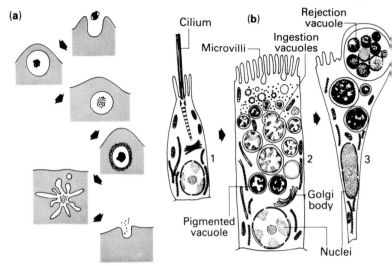

**Fig. 1–1** (a) Ingestion and intracellular digestion in the amoeba *Pelomyxa*. (b) Intracellular digestion in the digestive gland of a bivalve mollusc: (1) a young cell in its pre-absorptive stage; (2) a cell during absorption and digestion; (3) a cell during egestion.

endo-peptides), a collagenase, esterases (including acid phosphatase) and nucleases (both RNA-ase and DNA-ase).

The rhizopod protozoans, such as amoeba, are phagotrophic micro-carnivores ingesting other organisms into food vacuoles (Fig. 1–2a). Ciliates are the largest of the protozoans and in many ways foreshadow the complexity of metazoans. The ciliate *Paramecium* has a mouth, the cytostome, at the end of a cytopharynx towards which rows of food-collecting cilia converge. Food particles are impelled through this funnel by ciliary membranelles, enter digestive vacuoles which then pass through a regular cyclic pathway in the endoplasm, and the engested remains are finally expelled from a cytoproct (Fig. 1–2b, c). Carnivorous ciliates, such as *Didinium*, ingest paramecia several times larger than themselves by a cytostome set upon a pointed proboscis.

Intracellular digestion also occurs in the sponges. The flagellate choanocytes, or collar cells, in the inner walls of the sponge not only create water currents which carry food particles into the sponge, but also ingest the food particles. In the simple calcareous sponges the collars of the larger choanocyte cells are made up of microvilli which filter and trap particles which are then passed down the collar by protoplasmic streaming to be phagocytosed at the base. Intracellular digestion is initiated in vacuoles in the choanocytes, but the products are handed on to amoebocytes where digestion is completed and the products transferred throughout the colony (Fig. 1–2d, e).

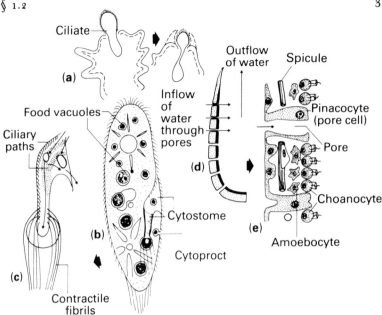

**Fig. 1–2**   Digestion in protozoans and sponges. (a) Ingestion of a ciliate by *Amoeba*. (b) Pathway of the food vacuoles through the endoplasm of *Paramecium*. (c) Detailed structure of the cytostome of *Paramecium*. (d) Vertical section through the body wall of a simple asconid sponge. (e) Details of the cellular structure of the body wall of an asconid sponge.

## 1.2   Extracellular digestion

In nearly all metazoan animals there is a permanent gut and so digestion becomes increasingly the work of enzymes secreted into the gut lumen. But in coelenterates, platyhelminthes, nemertines, polyzoans and many molluscs, annelids and echinoderms, the final stages of digestion long remain intracellular. The ultrastructure and activity of the cells of the digestive gland responsible for intracellular digestion in bivalve and gastropod molluscs have received special study. A sequence of stages can be identified, from uptake of particulate food, through digestion and assimilation, to egestion of residual matter into the gut lumen. The first stage is the maturation of small, undifferentiated cells with sparse flagella into mature absorbing cells with a zone of endocytotic vesicles beneath the fringe of microvilli. These vacuoles are converted to phagosomes by the acquisition of lysosomes which lie in the distal half of the cell. The vacuoles show progressive advances in digestion towards the cell base until at the final stage egestion vacuoles remain with unassimilable remains. The cell then rounds off at its free border and releases spherical fragments containing egestion vacuoles. These pass back into the stomach and are eliminated with the faeces. Lysosomes are also discharged in these fragments, and appear to initiate a new phase of extracellular digestion within the lumen (Fig. 1–1b).

## 1.3 The construction of the gut

The foods of animals range through virtually everything organic and so may vary enormously in difficulty of procuring and processing. Some foods, like egg yolk and honey, present both pure and highly concentrated nutriment. Some, like blood and milk and coelomic fluid, are nutritious but of inconveniently large volume. Others, such as plankton, require prolonged filtering and concentration, while still others, such as sand, mud and sawdust, are not only heavy and bulky but also very sparse in usable nutrients. The gut will naturally then vary greatly in its adaptations to the nature and bulk of different diets, but a general evolutionary pattern of gut development can be discerned.

In metazoans the different facets of the digestive process have become localized in different parts of the gut and specialized cells are grouped together. Enzymes are liberated to act outside the cell and this extracellular digestion is particularly appropriate for handling large prey. Nevertheless, some simple metazoans rely entirely on intracellular digestion. One of the most primitive flatworms, *Convoluta*, belonging to the order Acoela, has a gut with no internal lumen but a single aperture, the mouth, leading to a solid syncytium, or undifferentiated cell mass (Fig. 1–3b). This can be protruded somewhat like a giant pseudopodium and food is engulfed into vacuoles for intracellular digestion.

The triclad flatworm *Polycelis* also practises intracellular digestion. A long pharynx is inserted into the body of a bulky prey and food material is withdrawn in small fragments to be broken up by muscular contractions of the proboscis and thus prepared for intracellular digestion within the saccular diverticulate intestine (Fig. 1–3c). By contrast, the polyclad flatworm *Cycloporus*, which feeds on zooids of the compound ascidian *Botryllus*, everts a bell-shaped pharynx and sucks out whole zooids. These reach the gut intact, and are broken down entirely within the lumen by extracellular digestion (Fig. 1–3d).

*Hydra*, an example of the Coelenterata, has a simple gastrovascular or coelenteric cavity lined by gastrodermis (Fig. 1–3a). Water fleas ingested whole are broken down into small particles by extracellular digestion within four hours. Absorptive cells take up these particles into small vacuoles where digestion is completed. These same cells store reserve materials, and dispose of indigestible residues by cell fragmentation.

Although the gut of *Hydra* is simple the cells of the gastrodermis are diversified (Fig. 1–3f). The most numerous are digestive cells which ingest and intracellularly digest food particles. The organelles of these cells are comparable with protozoan food vacuoles and also with the organelles of the molluscan digestive cell (Fig. 1–1b). There are also gland cells of two types. One type secretes mucus to ease the passage of food through the

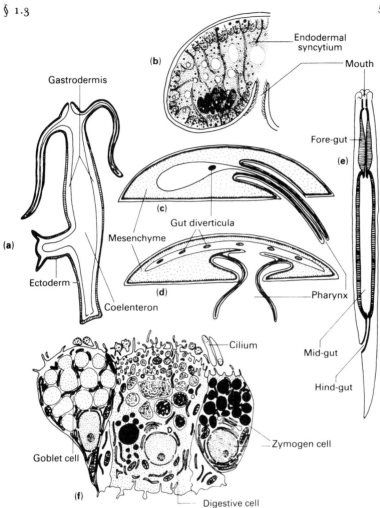

**Fig. 1–3** The structure of some primitive digestive systems. (a) *Hydra*. (b) Acoelan flatworm *Convoluta* with a syncytial endoderm. (c) Triclad flatworm *Polycelis*. (d) Polyclad flatworm *Cycloporus*. (e) A simple nematode illustrating gut structure with mouth and anus and the division of the gut into three parts. (f) The three types of cell found in the gastrodermis of *Hydra*.

oral opening and the other, the zymogen cell, releases enzymes for extracellular digestion.

In the Coelenterata and the Platyhelminthes the gut has only a single opening. The next stage in the functional separation of parts of the gut is seen in simple metazoans such as nemertines and pseudocoelomates. A second opening, the anus, is acquired and so the gut takes on the plan of a tube-within-a-tube. The three regions of the gut, fore-gut, mid-gut and hind-gut, that appeared early in evolution and appear constantly in all later metazoans, can be illustrated by a pseudocoelomate, the nematode (Fig. 1–3e). The fore-gut is a derivative of the embryonic stomodaeum and thus lined with ectoderm. It begins with a buccal or oral cavity, sometimes equipped with jaws or a piercing stylet, and leads through a muscular pharynx to an oesophagus of varying length. No enzymes are produced in the fore-gut, though secretions of the salivary glands released in the buccal cavity may become active here. The mid-gut is derived from endoderm and is a simple tube in nematodes, but it may variously be divided into stomach and intestine, and is the main site of enzyme secretion, digestion and absorption. In molluscs and non-insect arthropods the mid-gut develops a complex mass of diverticula, forming the digestive gland, and other invertebrates such as insects and starfish, have digestive caeca arising from the mid-gut. The hind-gut formed from the proctodaeum, and thus lined with ectoderm, generally has two regions, the colon and the rectum. Its function is to compact and discharge the faeces; in terrestrial animals large amounts of water are reabsorbed here.

Although vertebrates are the most complex metazoans there are close uniformities in gut structure throughout the group. The whole digestive process is now extracellular and except in a few special cases, such as the frog oesophagus, ciliary movement is superseded, and the gut is strongly muscular with rapid peristalsis. Most, but not quite all, vertebrates have a characteristic expanded stomach, separated by a sphincter, the pylorus, from the first part of the small intestine, the duodenum. The stomach constantly changes shape and churns and triturates food to reduce it to a milky chyme.

Peristaltic movements are regular and continuous, under the control of the autonomic nervous system. Peristalsis proceeds by contraction of circular muscle on the oral side and relaxation on the anal side of any stimulated point. Intestinal contents are thus forced towards the anus.

Extracellular digestion is not only rapid but allows division of labour. Different enzymes are produced in sequence by specialized cells, with the pH of the medium adjusted to their working range (Table 1). The vertebrate stomach is defined not by its recognizable form but by the possession of the enzyme pepsin, rarely found among invertebrates. The tubular gastric glands typically have three sorts of cell, goblet cells in the neck of the gland producing mucus, zymogen-type cells secreting pepsin, and parietal or oxyntic cells, distinguished by peculiar intracellular canaliculi, that secrete hydrochloric acid into the lumen (Fig. 1–4a, b, c).

Two organs, both unique to vertebrates, secrete into the duodenum shortly beyond the pylorus. The first, the pancreas, is of composite structure with both exocrine and endocrine portions. The endocrine portion is not directly concerned with digestion, but the exocrine part consists of acini lined with zymogen cells (Fig. 1–4f). These cells are traceable from the early digestive diverticulum of protochordates

(Amphioxus and some tunicates) and some lampreys (Fig. 1–4e) and correspond with the diffuse pancreatic follicles of teleost fish. In the elasmobranchs and all tetrapods, the compound pancreas is a massive gland, opening by a single duct into the duodenum.

Table 1 shows the sources and actions of enzymes including the pancreatic juice and the secretion of intestinal glands known as succus entericus. The pancreas also contributes sodium bicarbonate which reduces the acidity of the chyme received from the stomach.

The second organ, the liver, has many functions but enzyme production is not among them. Its alkaline secretion, the bile, contains bile salts, the breakdown products of haemoglobin, cholesterol and lecithin. The liver's main digestive role is the emulsification of fats by the bile salts, reducing their surface tension so as to break them up into a suspension of fine droplets. The distinctive histology of the liver is shown in Fig. 1–4d, g. Bile is manufactured by columns of cells, bathed by sinusoids, which are the ultimate small blood spaces. Blood passes centripetally through these from the interlobular portal vessels and hepatic arterioles, to the intralobular central vein, which drains back to the hepatic vein. Between the hepatic cells fine bile canaliculi lead centrifugally to the bile ducts.

The liver also has numerous metabolic functions: aminoacids taken up from the portal blood are deaminated, and the resultant —NH$_2$ converted to urea; absorbed carbohydrates are stored as glycogen; fat is accumulated as such, and metabolized; vitamin A is synthesized from carotene; the special phagocytic cells of Kuppfer remove foreign matter from the blood stream; old red blood cells are removed and, in the foetus, new ones contributed; the blood proteins, prothrombin and fibrinogen, are synthesized; and toxic substances such as alcohol are broken down and rendered harmless.

Intestinal digestion in the mammal leaves a fine milky suspension, chyle, whose contents are ready to be absorbed. The most active site of uptake is the small intestine beyond the duodenum, through the millions of small villi, which constantly contract and expand while bathed with digested food. Both monosaccharides and amino acids pass through the epithelium by active transport, against the diffusion gradient, into the blood plexus inside the villus, to be conducted to the portal circulation. Glucose transport is facilitated by conversion into a phosphate–sugar complex in the absorbing cells. Fats may be taken up by alternate routes: either, after hydrolysis to glycerol and fatty acids, by the portal circulation, or more generally, as a colloidal suspension of whole fat droplets, by the lacteals, which are the axial channels of the villi that lead ultimately to the thoracic duct of the lymphatic system (Fig. 1–4h, i).

The spacious colon has no digestive powers, but its epithelium contains abundant mucous glands. The gut contents remaining after digestion and absorption are concentrated by removal of water. In man, semi-solid faeces are produced after some 36 hours. With normal diet, little

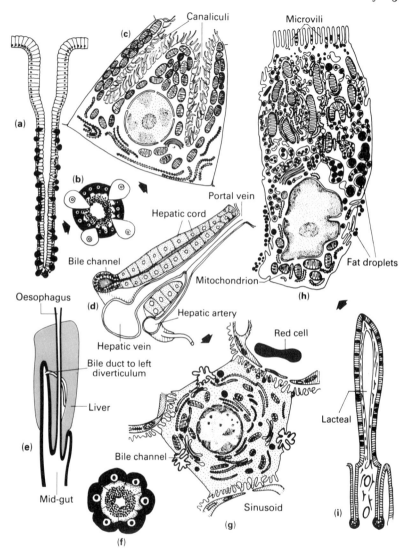

**Fig. 1–4** The fine structure of the vertebrate gut. (**a**) Mammalian gastric tubule showing the gland cells. (**b**) Cross-section of a mammalian gastric tubule. (**c**) Oxyntic cell from the mammalian gastric tubule showing the intracellular canaliculi. (**d**) Cord of hepatic cells and its associated vascular and bile channels. (**e**) Mid-gut of the larval lamprey showing the relationship between the mid-gut diverticula and the liver. (**f**) Cross-section of a pancreatic acinus from the teleost fish *Aldrichetta* showing the zymogen exocrine cells. (**g**) Mammalian liver cell. (**h**) Fat-absorbing cell of a mammalian villus. (**i**) Vertical section of a villus showing the lacteal vessel.

**Table 1** The sequence of digestive enzymes in the human gut. This enzyme complement is representative of that found in higher animals.

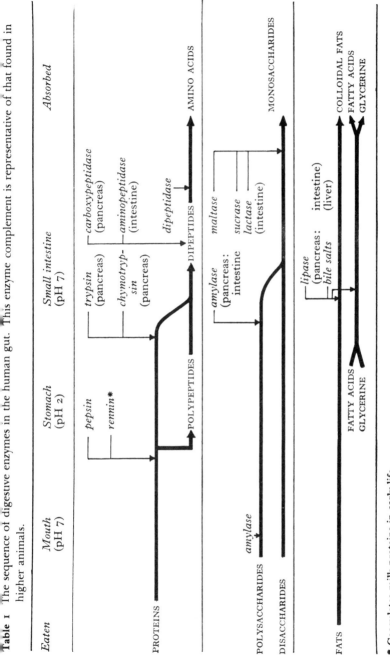

| Eaten | Mouth (pH 7) | Stomach (pH 2) | Small intestine (pH 7) | Absorbed |
|---|---|---|---|---|
| PROTEINS | | pepsin, rennin* → POLYPEPTIDES | trypsin (pancreas), chymotrypsin (pancreas) → ; carboxypeptidase (pancreas), aminopeptidase (intestine) → DIPEPTIDES; dipeptidase → | AMINO ACIDS |
| POLYSACCHARIDES, DISACCHARIDES | amylase → | | amylase (pancreas: intestine) → ; maltase, sucrase, lactase (intestine) → | MONOSACCHARIDES |
| FATS | | FATTY ACIDS GLYCERINE | lipase (pancreas: intestine), bile salts (liver) → | COLLOIDAL FATS, FATTY ACIDS, GLYCERINE |

* Coagulates milk proteins in early life.

undigested or indigestible food remains; faeces continue to be formed during starvation and contain chiefly the residues of bile and other internal secretions, leucocytes, sloughed-off epithelial cells, as well as vast numbers of bacteria, living and dead. They are coloured by stercobilin and other pigments of haemoglobin breakdown from the bile. Their unpleasant odour comes from the compounds indole and skatole, and $H_2S$, derived from the bacterial breakdown of sulphur-containing amino acids. Bacterial fermentation of carbohydrates also produces $CO_2$ and methane. The most vital role of the human colon is probably the synthesis of vitamins by its bacterial flora. Colon bacteria invade the infant shortly after birth, and remain important throughout life. Bodily production of the vitamin B complex (riboflavine, nicotinic acid, vitamin $B_{12}$ and vitamin K) is thereafter dependent on the superior synthetic ability retained by these symbionts.

### 1.4   A functional classification of guts

Although the preceding description reveals a progressive evolution in the complexity of gut structure and function, the remainder of this account will follow a simple functional classification. Lines of division will not follow animal groups but rather the food that animals ingest. Many animals of quite unrelated groups show convergence in the pattern and functions of the gut. This divergence is related to diet and so the lines of division can be made quite simple.

*Herbivores and omnivores*   The gut is here most generalized, with the fullest range of parts. In comparison with carnivores, the food is bulky and may have a large unassimilable component, though it is usually abundant and easy to obtain. The special category of *wood-eaters* is included here.

*Deposit feeders*   Ingesting large quantities of the soft substrate, the food being bulky, diffuse and of low nutritive content.

*Carnivores*   Living on a more concentrated and economic diet, often ingested at long intervals. Food may be of large bulk or small, but it is often hard to catch and there are many specializations for prehension, dismembering and swallowing.

*Filter feeders*   Continuously straining microscopic food from water by cilia and mucous films or screens of setae, often with elaborate devices for concentrating, sorting and transporting the fine food.

*Fluid feeders*   Taking liquids from plants or animals, generally with a piercing and sucking apparatus and some form of muscular pump. The rest of the gut is rather simply constructed, but with ample storage for the fluid meal.

In the following pages a brief survey will be made of each of these five divisions. Numerous examples, even within a single phylum, will be given. This is not profitless repetition, but is necessary to show the essential lesson of the gut which is the flexibility and adaptive resource it displays in nearly every animal group.

# 2 Herbivores and Omnivores

Though abundant and easy to procure, plant fodder contains stable structural polysaccharides very resistant to digestion. Few animals can by their own enzymes break down the beta-glucose linkages of which cellulose is built up. Instead they rely widely on symbiotic bacteria, ciliates or flagellates.

## 2.1 Cellulose digestion in ruminants, lagomorphs and macropods

In the ruminant mammals (e.g. cattle, sheep, antelope and deer), bacteria are of primary importance. The stomach and caecum (Fig. 2–1) are storage and fermentation chambers, equipped with a bacterial flora of facultative or obligate anaerobes that attack the food before its contact with digestive enzymes. Ciliate protozoans also live in the ruminant stomach. Bacterial digestion also occurs in the colon, not only in ruminants, but also in the horse and rabbit.

The gut bacteria break down 'difficult' compounds such as cellulose, which are converted in the stomach and elsewhere to volatile and absorbable fatty acids. Acetic acid can be formed *in vitro* by incubating a suspension of cotton wool cellulose with rumen contents at body temperature. Formic, acetic, propionic, butyric, succinic and lactic acids may be produced from various polysaccharides in the rumen and, contrary to popular belief, absorbed there. Blood from the rumen contains a high proportion of these acids, and in the sheep they account for about one quarter of the carbon assimilated from all carbohydrate sources. Carbon dioxide and methane are also produced by fermentation, and are either eructed or eliminated by the lungs. The water milieu and optimum pH in the bacterial chamber are maintained by copious saliva, rich in bicarbonate.

The ciliate protozoans of the rumen seem to play no part in cellulose digestion, although they do digest and assimilate starch. They also feed on the abundant bacteria and ultimately are themselves digested and so provide additional protein for their host. Some gut bacteria can also convert non-protein nitrogen into protein.

The rumen ciliates belong to the order Entodiniomorpha. Two examples are *Entodinium caudatum*, with a circlet of oral cilia and three posterior processes, the largest of which serves as a rudder, and *Epidinium ecaudatum*, with two tufts of immobile cirri at the oral end, and a so-called 'ventral skeletal plate' which is an important store of polysaccharides (Fig. 2–1g).

The ruminant stomach from the cow is illustrated in Fig. 2–1a, b. Only

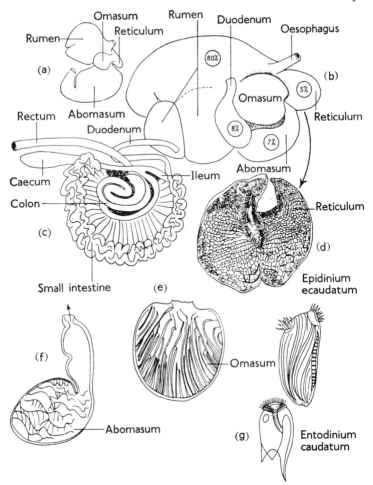

**Fig. 2–1** The ruminant stomach and its ciliates. (a) Stomach of newly-born calf. (b) Stomach. (c) Intestinal tract of adult ox. (d–f) Interior of reticulum, omasum and abomasum. (g) *Epidinium* and *Entodinium*.

the true stomach, or abomasum, has peptic glands and it opens straight to the pylorus. In the calf it is larger than all the rest, and provides the milk-coagulating enzyme rennin. The remaining three chambers have a horny lining epithelium and originate as oesophageal sacculations. They are the rumen or paunch; the reticulum or honeycomb (its lining is the source of honeycomb tripe); and the omasum, variously called the manifold, maniplies or psalterium, from its thin page-like folds of epithelium. Although small at birth, the rumen ultimately comes to account for 80% of the total stomach capacity. In feeding, grass passes first from the oesophagus into the recticulum where it is made up into small compacted balls of cud which are then returned to the mouth and chewed over at leisure. When re-swallowed, food enters the rumen, where it is subjected to bacterial digestion. The undigested contents pass on between the straining leaves of the omasum, and thence through the abomasum to the pylorus.

In the hares and rabbits (lagomorphs) the stomach is large and simple; but there is a long caecum with a well-developed vermiform appendix which harbours cellulose-digesting iodophile bacteria, as well as bacteria producing vitamin B (Fig. 2–2a). Hares and rabbits do not ruminate but re-ingest the faecal pellets; food thus passes through the gut twice and so is exposed twice to the digestive processes. There are no stomach ciliates, nor gastric uptake of volatile acids.

The macropods (kangaroos and wallabies) do not ruminate to any significant extent, but the large stomach (15% of the body weight when

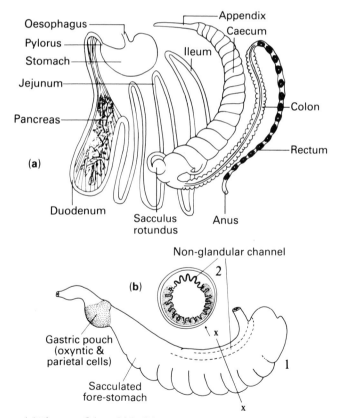

**Fig. 2–2** (a) The gut of the rabbit. (b) Kangaroo stomach: (1) stomach unfolded to display its regions; (2) cross-section (x—x) of the fore-stomach.

full) shows interesting parallels with that of the ruminants. The simple
stomach of the young in the pouch is transformed in the adult to a long
bag, deeply sacculated on its outer curvature (Fig. 2–2b); here it is lined
with non-glandular stratified epithelium, and corresponds to a reticulo-
rumen. Along its inner curvature a spiral groove directs non-fibrous food
to a thick-walled region, corresponding to the abomasum. The
epithelium here consists of parietal and pepsinogenic cells, and the pH
falls to 1.8–3.0. The sacculated chamber produces neither acid nor
enzymes, but has abundant cardiac mucous glands and dense
populations of symbionts (cellulolytic bacteria: $10^{10}$ $cm^{-3}$; protozoa: $10^7$
$cm^{-3}$). As well as gaseous $CO_2$ and hydrogen, this fermentation chamber
generates volatile fatty acids (acetic, propionic and butyric); their high
concentrations in the portal blood and reduced levels in the post-cardiac
stomach indicate that these acids are absorbed across the stomach wall
and metabolized by the liver to glucose. The symbionts utilize cellulose
for energy and obtain their nitrogen from recycling urea (as happens also
in sheep) while their phosphate requirement is met by recycling the large
quantities of RNA from bacteria digested in the abomasum and small
intestine.

## 2.2   Molluscs and echinoderms

Marine algae in shallow waters support many grazers and browsers,
chief among them some molluscs (gastropods and chitons) and the sea
urchins (Echinoidea). Algae contain a greater diversity of structural
polysaccharides than do land plants, and are energy-rich if they can be
depolymerized and the breakdown products thus made available. Red
algae contain agar (a polymer of galactose units) and iridophycin. Brown
algae contain algin (a polymer of mannose units), laminarin and
fucoidin.

Endogenous enzymes capable of splitting these substances are present
in many herbivores. The urchin *Strongylocentrotus* can degrade the
polysaccharides of brown algae. The giant chiton *Cryptochiton stelleri* can
digest fucoidin and laminarin, but not agar or iridophycin. Algin,
iridophycin and fucoidin are all attacked by the fore-gut enzymes of the
top-shell, *Tegula*. In numerous herbivorous molluscs enzymes have
been found which can split swollen cellulose fibres and water-soluble
sodium carboxymethylcellulose. In the land pulmonate *Helix*, where
cellulose digestion occurs, symbiotic bacteria are suspected to play a role.

The hall-mark of the molluscs is the abrading tooth ribbon, or radula,
lost only among the filtering bivalves. Primitive molluscan herbivores
such as ormers, top-shells, and turban-shells, have a wide radula which
sweeps delicately over irregular surfaces. In chitons, and in limpets and
periwinkles, the radula is narrower with stronger teeth and abrade
particles, including algal films and sporelings, from a hard substrate.

The two gastropod herbivores illustrated in Fig. 2–3 show contrasting designs for handling bulky plant food. In the grazing limpets (*Patella*) the strong radula is constantly worn away, and replaced from a coiled caecum almost twice the length of the body. The gut is much simplified from the primitive molluscan state. The oesophagus is the beginning of a wide storage tube, passing insensibly into the stomach and the first part of the intestine. The digestive gland produces a full enzyme complement and

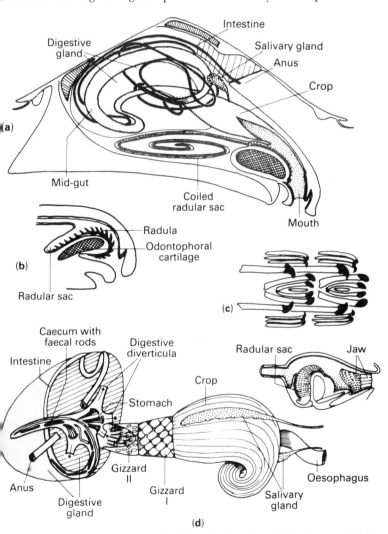

**Fig. 2–3** Herbivorous gastropods. (a) Sagittal section of the limpet, *Patella*, showing the gut. (b) Buccal mass of a generalized gastropod. (c) Radula teeth of the limpet, *Patella*. (d) Gut of the sea hare, *Aplysia*, with the buccal mass shown separately.

there are also two other enzyme sources, common in early prosobranchs, the salivary glands and the small oesophageal pouches, which secrete amylase. The intestine is long and many-looped and discharges a rope of bulky faeces into the mantle cavity behind the head.

In contrast, the opisthobranch sea hares (*Aplysia*) are browsers, cropping large pieces of succulent red, green and brown algae. The buccal cavity has strong lateral jaw plates and a small radula. But the fore-gut is highly complex, enlarged into a distensible crop, followed by two 'gizzards'. Of these, the first is an algal mincer, with heavy cuticular teeth, and in the second, the teeth are more slender and flexible and form a filter. Enzymes from the digestive gland circulate as food is shunted back and forth through the stomach, gizzards and crop. The partly digested fluid contents of the stomach are forced by pressure of the stomach walls into the digestive diverticula, for phagocytosis and intracellular digestion. Indigestible residues pass into a narrow caecum of the stomach where faecal rods are prepared.

The land pulmonates (*Helix*) are also browsers, and bite off their prolific supply of plant food with the radula and the single median jaw. The radula is a broad ribbon with thousands of small, unspecialized teeth. The crop is simplified into a long cistern, continuous with the stomach, through which a sherry-coloured digestive fluid ebbs and flows.

The Echinoderms have a novelty of structure and design which is typified by Aristotle's lantern; this is a unique abrading organ, which is to the regular echinoids what the radula is to the molluscs (Fig. 2–4). It forms a cluster of five jaw-pieces, converging like chisels through the opened mouth. At the roof of the lantern these are linked by alternating pieces called *rotulae*, overlaid by five radial *compasses*. Radial jaw retractor muscles can pivot the lantern tip in any direction from the mouth; other muscles coordinate the opening and closing of the teeth, and also up and down movements of the lantern roof that circulate respiratory water in the surrounding coelom.

Like the limpets, many of the regular echinoids occupy a home scar, and make wide grazing forays cropping not only growing algae but small sessile animals, such as barnacles, polyzoans and hydroids, as well as organic debris. Food is carried by peristalsis up through the muscular oesophagus. Water passes in too, but short-circuits the stomach and arrives directly in the intestine by way of a narrow parallel by-pass, the siphon.

The stomach is a spacious thin-walled tube, making a clockwise circuit, attached in short festoons to the test. The intestine returns in the reverse direction and ascends to the anus. The stomach is the seat of digestion and absorption and is an area of intense phagocytic activity. The granular cells of the epithelium secrete a full complement of enzymes. In addition several sorts of amoebocyte regularly cross the stomach wall. Red colourless and green 'granulocytes' cluster around food particles within the lumen, to absorb and distribute soluble nutriment. Other

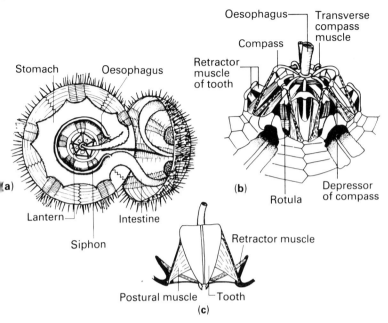

**Fig. 2–4**   The gut of the sea urchin, *Echinus esculentus*. (a) The test of the urchin has been divided into two hemispheres to show the whole gut. (b) Details of Aristotle's lantern and its musculature. (c) Vertical division of Aristotle's lantern to show the teeth.

ameobocytes ('agranulocytes') phagocytose particulate matter for intracellular digestion.

Loaded amoebocytes migrate to the lacunae of the haemal system, which spreads over the gut, and accumulate in the main haemal depots. Such engulfment by wandering amoebocytes is an efficient method of non-localized intracellular digestion. The haemal system of echinoderms differs from a true blood system in that nutritive and excretory materials are transported by migratory cells in strands of soft tissue, not in fluids pumped through vessels. The haemal system also absorbs much water from the stomach.

The intestine and rectum conduct undigested waste by peristalsis to the anus, where loose, rather incoherent strings of faeces are discharged.

## 2.3   The insect gut

The insects are small persistent and prolific land arthropods. In addition to flying power, and specialized life histories, they owe much of their success to enzymes capable of splitting numerous unpromising foods, including, it has been noted, 'such unusual materials as horn, fur, feathers, cork, pepper, beeswax and cured tobacco, which are the exclusive choices of certain species'.

Early generalized insects, such as the Orthoptera, are herbivores and omnivores, and a suitable starting point for a study of the insect gut is the grasshopper or the cockroach (Fig. 2–5).

The fore-gut is derived from stomodaeum and is thus lined with cuticle. The salivary glands open into the pharynx and saliva serves to moisten the food and lubricate the mouthparts, as well as providing a

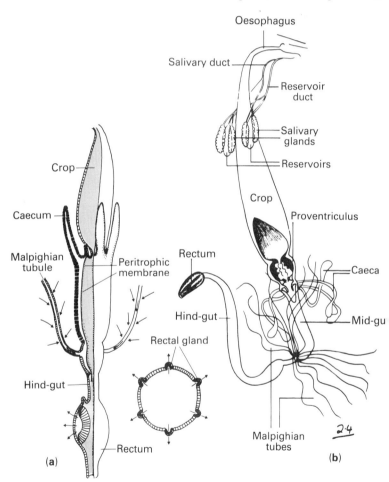

**Fig. 2–5**   (a) Diagrammatic vertical section of the gut of the grasshopper *Anacridium*, showing the peritrophic membrane and the movements of water in through the Malpighian tubules and out through the rectal glands. (b) Gut of the cockroach, *Periplaneta americana*, dissected to show the interior of the proventriculus.

powerful amylase and invertase which initiate the digestion of starch and disaccharides. The narrow oesophagus opens into a long fusiform crop, which is an important seat of digestion both by salivary enzymes and by mid-gut enzymes which are carried forward. Little glucose or water is absorbed in the crop, but olive oil may pass across its lining.

Behind the crop the fore-gut lining of some Orthoptera is massively thickened to form a spherical proventriculus or gizzard (Fig. 2–5b). This can vary in different insects from a muscular sphincter to a powerful triturating chamber, and in the cockroach has six strong, radially inserted teeth. Beyond the teeth, a corresponding row of hairy cushions serves as a food strainer. Crushed contents are returned to the crop for further digestion, while the fluid products finally seep through the filter to the mid-gut.

In the mid-gut the epithelium bears no lining cuticle as such, but in almost all insects is kept free from abrasion by the gut contents, not by a mucous lining as in vertebrates, but by a delicate detached sheath of chitin and protein known as the peritrophic membrane. This special structure is very permeable to molecules, keeping back only dyes of large molecular weight and allowing enzymes and the products of digestion to pass without hindrance. In the cockroach the peritrophic membrane is produced directly by the underlying cells in thin concentric sheets, the inner layers being periodically passed backwards as investments of the faeces.

The fore-gut lining projects into the mid-gut, directing the contents into the cylinder formed by the peritrophic membrane. The surface of the mid-gut is increased by the outgrowth of five or six long blunt-tipped caeca near its anterior end, and the peritrophic membrane simply spans the mouth of these (Fig. 2–5). Secretion and absorption within the mid-gut and its caeca are generally carried out by the same cells, which in the cockroach undergo alternate phases of activity. The cells may also store absorbed or metabolized substances, such as fat droplets after a sugar meal. Numerous enzymes are contributed by the mid-gut cells including protease, lipase and maltase. With the acid crop contents, the salivary amylase works best at a pH of 5.9, and the mid-gut proteases at 7.5, though they may function efficiently well over to the acid side of neutrality. The so-called 'protease' has several components, a trypsin (though never a pepsin) acting on whole proteins and peptidases splitting the later products, including amino-polypeptidase active at the $NH_2$ linkage, a carboxypolypeptidase attacking —COOH groups and a dipeptidase hydrolyzing all dipeptides. While the proteinases are active in the lumen, the peptidases seem to be concentrated within the cells.

At the boundary of the mid-gut with the hind-gut a series of threadlike excretory organs, the Malpighian tubules, discharge their contents into the lumen. Insinuating their way through the whole visceral mass and among the lobules of the fat body, these organs are finer and more numerous in the Orthoptera than in most other insects. Their chief product is uric acid.

The hind-gut, like the fore-gut, has a thin lining cuticle, but it is readily permeable to water. It begins with a long and narrow colon, opening into a short, wide rectum, where the lining cells tend to separate into six pads or folds known as rectal glands. In the Orthoptera the faeces become progressively drier as they pass back and the rectal glands play a large part in the absorption of water. Dry faecal pellets are produced after 9–13 hours. They are invested with peritrophic membrane which is drawn backwards by spinules on the hind-gut cuticle.

## 2.4   Wood-borers and swallowers

A wide variety of carbohydrates contribute to the composition of wood. Lignin (some 18–38% of the total) is, as far as is known, never digested. Cellulose (40–62% of the total) is, however, frequently broken down to its assimilable glucose units. In many wood-eating insects bacteria are responsible for the breakdown of cellulose. Some cellulose-digesting bacteria present in rotting wood may continue their work after ingestion, and some wood-boring lamellicorn beetle larvae have enlargements of the hind-gut which act as fermentation chambers in which bacterial action is fostered. The wood-eating cockroach, *Panesthia*, keeps cellulose-decomposing bacteria in the crop.

Certain species of cockroach, and also the termites (Isoptera) rely heavily on a diet of wood. In the cockroach *Cryptocercus*, and in the termites (with the exception of the 'highest' family, the Termitidae), the hind-gut is enlarged to form a pouch with a greater capacity than all of the rest of the gut (Fig. 2–6a). This chamber contains a teeming population of large and complex flagellates, which belong to the order Hypermastigina and are frequently packed in a seemingly pure mass. Some of their characteristic shapes are illustrated in Fig. 2–6d, e. *Lophomonas* is typical of the common cockroach, and *Trichomonas* and the very large *Trichonympha* are found in the termite gut. Gut flagellates ingest fine particles of wood and different species might play different roles in digesting the various constituents. It has also been suggested that the digestion of wood is carried out by symbiotic bacteria contained within the flagellates. Termites can live on a diet of pure cellulose if they are not deprived of their flagellates by starvation, or exposure to high temperatures or high oxygen tension. In *Zootermopsis*, some two-thirds of the material absorbed from wood is rendered assimilable by flagellates.

Two widespread marine borers in wooden ships and piles, the shipworm *Teredo* and the isopod *Limnoria*, make efficient use of cellulose as food. The gut of *Limnoria* is exceptional in having no microorganisms, but the enzymes of its mid-gut diverticula break down wood cellulose, filter-paper, cellophane and carboxymethylcellulose, as well as starch and glycogen. Half the cellulose and almost all the polyuronide hemicellulose are removed from the wood during digestion. Proteins appear to be supplied from the fungi that infect woods exposed to sea-water; *Limnoria* can survive neither on sterile wood nor in sterile sea-water.

The highly aberrant bivalve mollusc *Teredo* also has a dietary supplement as it continues to filter plankton during the 'quiescent' phases that alternate with active movements of shell adduction and wood-boring. Wood chips are freely ingested through the mouth, and stored in a long gastric appendix that converts a spasmodic flow into a steady stream for digestion. The crystalline style (see p. 39) is smaller than in other bivalves, and the right and left gastric caeca have openings to two sorts of digestive gland tubules. In the first, filtered food is ingested, as in other bivalves. The second forms a loose syncytium, capable of phagocytosing the wood particles, which are nearly always found in the lumina, being directed there by the sorting cilia of the stomach (Fig. 2–6b, c).

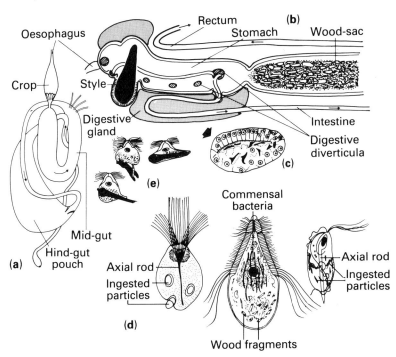

**Fig. 2–6** The gut structure of some wood-eaters. (**a**) Gut of the termite, *Eutermes*, showing the rectal pouch. (**b**) Longitudinal section of the alimentary tract of the shipworm, *Teredo navalis*. (**c**) Tubule of the digestive gland of *Teredo*, showing phagocytosed wood particles. (**d**) Flagellates symbiotic in the gut of insects: (1) *Lophomonas blattarum* (20 μ) from the cockroach; (2) *Trichonympha collaris* (250 μ) and (3) *Trichomonas termopsidis* (30 μ) from *Zootermopsis*. (**e**) *Trichonympha* ingesting wood particles.

# 3 Deposit Feeders

## 3.1 Introduction

The most bulky and apparently un-nutritive of diets are those obtained by animals ingesting the whole substrate. These unselective deposit feeders are in fact a smaller class than has commonly been thought; almost always some selection is made of the richer organic material at the surface. Thus the lug-worms, *Arenicola*, appear to swallow entire sand, but get their chief food from the conical head-shaft of their burrow which fills with subsiding deposits from the surface layer. This is rich in diatoms, dinoflagellates, protozoa and much organic debris.

The sand-burrowing worms of the genus *Ophelia* have similar feeding habits. The crowded population of an intertidal beach can pass the whole top 15 cm through their guts in a couple of seasons. The actively burrowing worm, *Sipunculus*, ingests the surface sand with its eversible fringed proboscis. Acorn worms, *Balanoglossus*, also pass voluminous sand castings, yet their feeding does not involve merely the automatic swallowing of sand as they burrow. Glands on the proboscis and collar secrete not only mucus but an amylolytic enzyme, and collected food particles are carried by cilia from the collar to the mouth. Some food is also filtered by the gill slits from the powerful respiratory current in a manner foreshadowing the ciliary feeding of protochordates (see p. 35).

Sea cucumbers or holothurians push the surface deposits into their mouths by means of the circlet of oral tentacles. Largest and most numerous on the coral sand flats of tropical reefs, they feed continuously, passing prolific cylinders and coils of sandy faeces. The first portion of the gut, the tubular stomach, has muscular walls but no particular organs of trituration. Undoubtedly particles are subjected to mutual abrasion and comminution as they rub together during passage through the gut. The walls of the long intestine are surprisingly delicate and thin, and in the sand-burrowing holothurian, the worm-like *Synapta* (Fig. 3–1c), the gut and body wall together resemble merely a transparent sausage casing stretched over the contained column of sand particles. In the sea cucumber the cloaca functions as a respiratory organ, taking in by muscular contractions a constant flow of water to fill the internal gill system of the 'respiratory trees' (Fig. 3–1d).

## 3.2 Deposit-feeding worms

The gut of the lugworm, *Arenicola*, a deposit-feeding worm is shown in Fig. 3–1a. The lugworm ingests by everting and withdrawing its short,

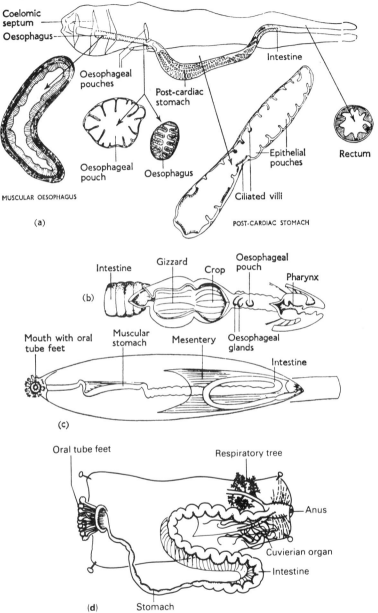

**Fig. 3–1** (a) Gut of the lug-worm, *Arenicola marina*, with anterior body septa and transverse sections of the successive regions. (b) Anterior part of the gut of the earthworm, *Lumbricus terrestris*. (c) Synaptid holothurian dissected to show the first part of the gut. (d) Gut and associated organs of the sea-cucumber, *Holothuria forskali*.

rounded proboscis. The swallowings are stored temporarily in the short oesophagus and, aided by rhythmic contractions of the body wall, it is this section of the gut that initiates the movement of the food. Two pear-shaped oesophageal pouches open just before the stomach, producing a watery secretion with some amylase. Mixed with this the food passes back in a more fluid state to the stomach, where the gut dilates and its wall is distended with close-set pouches or saccules, bright yellow from chloragogenous tissue. Patches of cilia in the stomach keep the contents well mixed, bringing them in contact with the epithelium of the pouches and with the ciliated, cup-shaped villi which are a feature of the wall between the pouches. The pH within the stomach is depressed to 5.4–6.0 and the principal enzymes are protease and amylase.

It has been estimated that about 96% of the material swallowed is inorganic and of no nutritive value whatever. Large total quantities must thus be put through, and maximum extraction employed; the straight gut of a narrow worm offers little storage space and quick elimination is required to make way for the introduction of fresh swallowings. Faeces are rhythmically voided some 45 minutes after ingestion and, while food is in the stomach, effective means are employed to glean its sparse nutritive content. Enzymes act extracellularly and at the same time particles are engulfed phagocytically by the epithelial cells of the stomach wall. At the base of the epithelium these are taken up by coelomic cells which may carry material into the blood stream or the coelom.

In the intestine, water is absorbed, firmer faeces are produced and temporarily stored in the rectum as cylinders coated and lightly bound with mucus.

In selective deposit feeders and ciliary feeders there are complex adaptations for sorting and manipulating the smaller but richer particle flow. In massive deposit swallowers, where the bulk of food is too great, or its nutritive content too sparse, all expedients for sorting have been abandoned.

## 3.3   Earthworms

The most important terrestrial substrate swallowers are the earthworms of the Lumbricidae, made famous by the studies of Charles Darwin. Where the soils are over-compact the earthworms certainly burrow by eating their way through them, though not all earthworm species have the same feeding habits. *Lumbricus terrestris* most commonly forms a U-shaped burrow from which it protrudes the front end to feed from the surface. Large fragments of dead or fresh organic matter, especially leaves, are drawn down into the burrow. These are moistened in patches by a secretion of alkaline reaction containing an amylase by which starch grains are sometimes externally digested. Pieces may then be torn off the moistened leaf between the prostomium and the lower border of the mouth, or withdrawn into the mouth by the sucking action of the muscular pharynx. In addition, much earthy material is swallowed, of particle size up to 2 mm.

The gut of the earthworm (Fig. 3–1b) begins with a thick-walled dilatable pharynx, having a narrow cavity and strong extrinsic muscles running to the body wall. Behind the pharynx is a short oesophagus into which open, in *Lumbricus*, three pairs of lime-secreting diverticula (one of oesophageal pouches, two of oesophageal 'glands'). Behind the oesophagus the gut widens to a muscular, pear-shaped crop; this storage chamber opens in turn into a spherical gizzard with a strong endowment of muscle. Here, no doubt, as probably elsewhere, particle size is reduced by rubbing and abrasion. The gizzard leads back into the long, straight intestine, with its secreting and absorbing surface increased by a large typhlosolar fold. Movement of gut contents is mainly peristaltic, though the lining cells are ciliated and interspersed with mucus goblets.

The faeces are voided in *Lumbricus*, though not in all earthworms, in the well-known surface casts. Charles Darwin calculated that the cast-making earthworms bring to the surface 2–60 tonnes per hectare per year by their feeding activities. In soils of good pasture land there is commonly a stone-free layer 10–20 cm deep and it has been estimated that the top 10 cm pass through the alimentary tract of earthworms in $11\frac{1}{2}$ years where there is a high population. By selecting and triturating organic particles, the worms bring about a large and intimate mixture of new organic debris with the soil. In comparison with the soil, worm casts have more total and more nitrate nitrogen, more total and exchangeable calcium, more exchangeable potassium and magnesium, more available phosphate, more organic carbon and a greater base exchange capacity. The casts are also more nearly neutral in reaction than the original surface soil, sometimes 75% more so. This is apparently due to the alkaline secretions of the gut as a whole, rather than to the particular output of the calciferous glands which produce crystals of largely inactive calcite and are said to be primarily excretory in their role.

# 4 Carnivores

## 4.1 Carnivores in various phyla

The rewards of a carnivorous life are nutritively rich. Muscle and other proteins are among the most compact and economic of foods; but, easy though it may be to assimilate, the single unit of animal food frequently requires great expenditure of energy to catch and immobilize. If the prey unit is too small it is scarcely worth the expense of catching; being of economic catch size, it is certain to be bulky to swallow, and hence many carnivores take intermittent, over-large meals, and are apt to enter upon a quiescent period of digestion.

The problem of bulk may be overcome in one of three ways: by a mouth and fore-gut distensible and capacious enough to take in a meal at one massive swallowing; by teeth employed not only for prehension but for shearing and dismembering; and by reducing the prey to a liquid form with enzymes acting outsde the body, so that the gut is presented simply with a rich protein broth.

In contrast with problems of pursuit, sedentary food may be difficult of access through being enclosed in heavy shells or exoskeletons. Such hard casings may be crushed by toothed or muscular gizzards after swallowing whole, or, with more subtlety, the shells may be bored through or entered by narrow chinks and the food taken out in small fragments. The most important group of externally digesting carnivores are undoubtedly the Arachnida, which are so uniformly adapted for this habit that they may best be considered among 'Fluid Feeders'.

The earliest metazoan carnivores massively swallow the prey, just as an *Amoeba* or a carnivorous ciliate will engulf a living flagellate. The Coelenterata, nearly all carnivores, reduce the prey to possession by grappling it with the tentacles after contact with stinging cells or nematoblasts. The food is then pushed or held against the mouth with the tentacles and engulfed by the contraction of the circular pharyngeal muscles. The whole body cavity or *coelenteron* is generally held to serve as a 'gut' but in the largest of the polyps, the anemones, a special investment of active digestive epithelium closes around the body of the prey. After feeding *Calliactis parasitica* with coloured gelatin blocks, the food bolus below the stomodaeum was found to be completely invested with closely adhering mesenteric filaments (Fig. 4–1a, b). These structures are the glandular edges of the radial folds or mesenteries that divide up the coelenteron; they are clad with both secreting and absorbing cells, and move actively over the bolus, each lifting off and being replaced with another as its cells become engorged with food. Secretion of a powerful

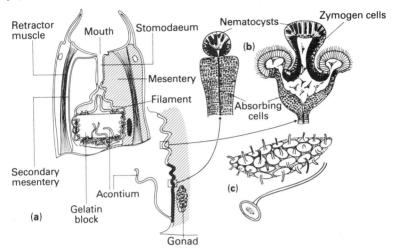

**Fig. 4–1** (a) Diagrammatic vertical section of an anemone fed with a gelatin block to show the disposition of the mesenteric filaments. (b) Histological detail of the ciliated and glandular portions of the filament. (c) Trumpet mouths of gastrozooids of *Physalia* investing the body of a captured fish; one mouth is shown enlarged.

protease, stimulated by protein food, initiates contact digestion at the epithelial surface. The food mass shrinks and dissolves as the filaments press upon it, and waste is defecated in a compact mucus-coated pellet by contractile movements of the column. The remainder of the coelenteron may simultaneously act as a respiratory organ, water entering it freely by the ciliated gutters or *siphonoglyphs* running down either side of the inturned sleeve of the mouth, or stomodaeum.

An analogous temporary 'stomach' of separate digestive units encloses the food of some siphonophores, such as the Portuguese man-o'-war, *Physalia*. Prey captured with the long fishing tentacles, or dactylozooids, is drawn up and held close beneath the float. It is then invested by the trumpet mouths of 100 or more gastrozooid polyps, adhering like little suckers and pouring upon it a supply of proteolytic enzyme (Fig. 4–1c).

The primitive gut of the free-living flatworms, with no separate anus, has already been described (p. 4); the planarians have three blind intestinal branches, and the polyclads show repeatedly branching outgrowths from a central stomach.

The proboscis-worms (phylum Nemertea) were the first metazoans to acquire a separate anus. The gut is a long featureless tube and its most characteristic organ is the proboscis; this lies in a muscular proboscis sheath running along the dorsal side of the gut, and opening separately above the mouth. The proboscis is rapidly eversible, being shot out by the pressure of fluid in the sheath to a length sometimes more than that of the body. It entwines round the prey and immobilizes it with mucus or other secretions, to be then conveyed to the mouth and swallowed entire.

The same mode of ingestion is practised by carnivorous polychaete worms such as *Nereis*, *Nephthys*, *Glycera* and *Eunice*, all of which have a muscular introvert or pharynx, with its eversible lining equipped with small teeth. In the sea-mouse, *Aphrodite*, the pharynx is a heavily muscular tube with a narrow lumen, and serves as a gizzard for crushing animal food.

Among the carnivorous echinoderms, the starfishes (Asteroidea) frequently digest the prey externally by everting the stomach over it and pouring out a supply of proteolytic enzymes (Fig. 4–2). The long-armed

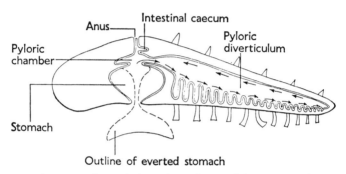

**Fig. 4–2**   Diagrammatic vertical section of a starfish, *Asterias*, showing the regions of the gut and its diverticula.

Asteroidea feed chiefly upon bivalve molluscs. The shell is wrenched open by the suction power of the multiple tube feet, applied relentlessly until the adductor muscle of the bivalve relaxes from fatigue. The stomach is then extruded as a thin collapsible bag and inserted into the slightly gaping shell; it can be stretched to a great capacity and is finally withdrawn through the mouth, filled with liquefied and partly digested food. Most of the space within the central disc of the star is filled by this bag. Opening from it above is a smaller pyloric chamber with a short, narrow intestine leading directly upwards to the aboral surface. Digestion is completed by the enzymes from the pyloric caeca, a pair of long, much-folded glandular diverticula extending into each of the five, or more, arms. Enzymes are carried to the stomach by outward ciliary currents while along the opposite wall, ingoing currents bring soluble material into the caeca for absorption. Large indigestible waste is voided through the mouth, small fragments through the anus.

Three gastropods adapted to swallow whole prey are shown in Fig. 4–3. *Philine* crushes bivalve shells with a box-like, heavily toothed gizzard; *Testacella* swallows earthworms by its massive, sharp-toothed odontophore (shown fully everted); and *Gymnodoris* has a distensible buccal mass, modified for engulfing other nudibranchs.

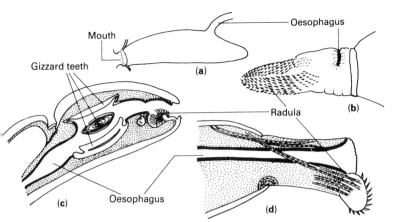

**Fig. 4–3**  The interior gut structure of some gastropods adapted for massive swallowing. (a) Buccal mass of the slug *Testacella*. (b) Fully extended odontophore of *Testacella*. (c) Tectibranch *Philine* showing the calcified gizzard teeth. (d) Everted odontophore and radula of the nudibranch *Gymnodoris*.

The cone shells are noted for the sudden capture and swallowing of moving prey, including blennies, gobies and other small fish. A neurotoxin from the salivary glands is injected into the prey by the special harpoon-like radular teeth. There is no odontophore, and the radula caecum is bent at a sharp angle; each limb contains a sheaf of slender teeth, barbed at the tips. The shaft forms a partly closed tube, conveying the poison from the opening of the salivary duct (Fig. 4–4). The toxin of the geography cone (*Conus geographus*) and several others has at times proved fatal to man.

The quarry is located by the chemoreceptors of the osphradium, leading the cone to crawl towards it and 'cover' it with the poised proboscis. With each successful strike a single harpoon is shot out and lodged. Its struggles quelled, the whole fish is smoothly engulfed into the distensible proboscis sheath. Rapid proteolytic digestion follows as the first part of the prey is passed into the oesophagus, and with the progress of digestion the whole mass is softened and received into the fore-gut.

The most prodigious swallowers are probably to be found among some of the deep-sea fish. In the small black lantern fish *Melanocoetus* (Fig. 4–5a) the wide vertical mouth and the great bag of the throat dominate the whole design of the body. The gulper eels, *Eurypharynx*, have the jaws grotesquely underslung; the mouth opens chiefly by the dropping of the lower jaw with its own weight, and the closing musculature is also weak. But the mouth forms a huge receptacle that can be widened by spreading the jaw framework sideways to engulf prey far larger than the predator.

A still more bizarre design of the mouth is shown by the deep-water stomatoid fish, *Malacosteus indicus* (Fig. 4–5b). The jaws are slender struts

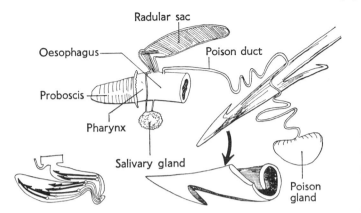

**Fig. 4–4** Anterior part of gut of *Conus striatus*. The terminal part of a single tooth is shown superimposed with, below, an enlargement of the grooved barb. Lower left is a diagram of the teeth in the radular sac.

with the angle carried well back below the body. By the contraction of special muscle bands they can be swung open and forward with great speed, and the lower jaw can snap suddenly at a passing animal, like the mask of a predatory dragon-fly. The sharp fang teeth strike into the prey as the jaw is swung backwards. It is then thrown into the spacious framework of the mouth as the jaws snap shut. The skin of the whole back and floor of the mouth has disappeared, removing a water resistance that would be too great for the closing of the jaws. The only framework behind

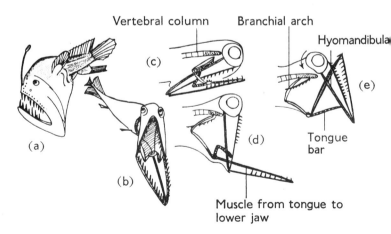

**Fig. 4–5** Some large-mouthed deep sea fish: (**a**) the angler fish, *Melanocoetus cirrifer*; (**b**) *Malacosteus indicus* with the gape fully open; (**c–e**) stages in the opening and closing of the jaws.

the jaws is of the lateral hyoid bones and the narrow muscle band to the interangle of the mandibles.

## 4.2   Cephalopoda

These molluscs are pre-eminent for their high tempo of life, both in their jet locomotion and their fast capture and digestion of food. In the squid, *Loligo*, taking small fish, or the cuttle-fish, *Sepia*, feeding on shrimps, the prey is secured by the lightning extension of the two tentacular arms, normally kept ensheathed. The octopus by contrast pounces on crabs and similar prey with its outspread arms and inter-arm web.

In all cephalopods the prey is held against the mouth by the circlet of suckered arms and its struggles are stilled by the injection of a toxin from the posterior salivary glands. In the octopus this contains tyramine, octopamine and hydroxytryptamine, which have a powerful effect on the nervous system. The food is bitten into small pieces by the horny parrot-like beak, aided by strokes of the small radula. Powerful salivary proteases are injected from the salivary glands and the food is reduced to a semi-pulpy condition before being cleaned out from the exoskeleton and carried down the oesophagus to the stomach (Fig. 4–6d).

The gut of *Loligo* is shown in Fig. 4–6a. The oesophagus is narrow and muscular and the stomach is a large contractile bag, capable of vigorous peristalsis. It serves as a gizzard where food is thoroughly churned and subjected to preliminary digestion. A narrow isthmus from the stomach leads to the caecum, a thin-walled sac forming an annexe to the ducts from the digestive glands and also leading to the opening of the intestine. The Cephalopoda possess two sorts of digestive gland, known rather inappropriately as 'liver' and 'pancreas'. Both produce proteolytic and amylolytic enzymes. The secretion of the pancreas is the first to become active, being driven into the stomach from the caecum where it has been stored.

After early digestion for an hour or more in the stomach, food is released in instalments to the caecum where it remains up to 4 hours. Digestion is completed by the action of 'liver' secretion. Resistant solid particles are all the while removed from the caecum to the intestine by the action of the ciliated organ of the caecal wall. This is a set of converging folds and leaflets with currents directed towards the intestine. With the nutrient fluid cleared of all solid remains, absorption of soluble products takes place in the large, thin-walled caecal sac. At intervals the remaining residue in the caecum is voided to the intestine (Fig. 4–6a).

An intricate arrangement of valves and channels keeps these different functions segregated and properly phased. The efficiency of the cephalopod gut lies in its rapidity of digestive action; this can be renewed whenever food is available, while the processing of a previous meal is allowed to go on at the same time.

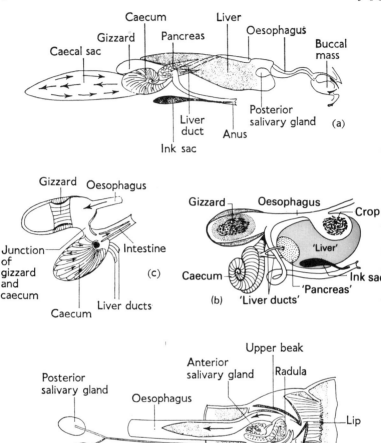

**Fig. 4–6** The cephalopod gut. (a) Gut of *Loligo*. (After BIDDER, A. M. (1950). *Quart. J. Micr. Sci.*, **91**, 1.) (b) Schematic section of the gut of *Octopus* with the buccal mass removed. (c) Diagram of the stomach of *Sepia*, in longitudinal section. (d) Buccal mass and associated glands in *Sepia*.

## 4.3 Crustacea

The largest and most advanced of the Crustacea, the crayfish and crabs and lobsters, form a contrast in many ways to the Cephalopoda. Though some of them are fleet of foot, they are all benthic rather than fast-swimming, and they feed on an indiscriminate range of slow prey. Small animals, such as worms and molluscs, and dead tissues are pushed to the mouth by a complex battery of limbs and are finally seized and ingested by the heavy mandibles. The fore-gut incorporates a complex system of mincers and filters; the mouth parts are an apparatus designed for thoroughness rather than speed.

As in all arthropods, the crustacean gut begins with a large chitinized stomodaeum and terminates with a proctodaeum, both ectodermal. In between, and derived from the endoderm, is the mid-gut or mesenteron. A short oesophagus leads directly up to the stomach, which is the site of internal trituration, pressing and filtering the food in preparation for absorption by the digestive gland. Forming part of the stomodaeum, the stomach has a chitinous lining throughout its two parts, the larger 'cardiac' chamber in front and the smaller 'pyloric' chamber behind. Near the junction of these chambers, the stomach roof is occupied by a gastric mill, a set of lining plates and heavy teeth formed by the local thickening of the chitin. The pyloric chamber incorporates a mid-gut filter, a filter press and a gland filter; the last-named guards on either side the aperture of the digestive gland, which is a soft and very extensive yellow-brown mass, built up of fine tubules packed around and behind the stomach. The crustacean digestive gland, like that of the Mollusca, is not only absorptive but secretory; its epithelium has, however, separate

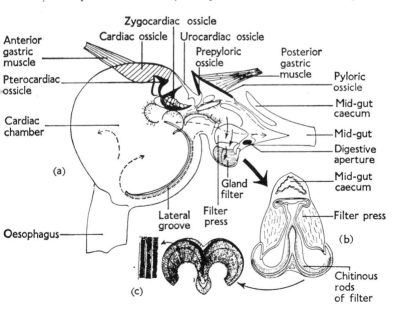

**Fig. 4–7**   The stomach of the Norway lobster, *Nephrops norvegicus*. (a) The cardiac and pyloric chambers in sagittal section. (b) Cross-section of the region of the filter press and gland filter. (c) Detail of the gland filter (removed) and of its chitinous rods. (After YONGE, C. M. (1924). *J. exp. Biol.*, **1**, 343.)

cells subserving each role. In the crayfish, proteolytic, amylolytic and lipolytic enzymes are passed outwards from the follicles of the gland to flow back along the ventral pyloric channels to the cardiac chamber. They enter this region at either side along the comb-fringed ventrolateral grooves, continuous with the ventral channels. Extracellular digestion takes place here and most of the soluble products flow back through the gland filter and into the digestive diverticula for absorption. A small and subsidiary amount of absorption occurs in the straight mid-gut, or in the short caeca from it.

The ossicles of the gastric mill are shown in Fig. 4–7. The prepyloric and pyloric plates are freely hinged and, by the action of anterior and posterior gastric muscles attaching to the stomach, the median tooth and the two strong lateral teeth are brought together, breaking up anything lying between them. The anterior part of the pyloric chamber is guarded from the cardiac chamber by a massive cardiopyloric valve, covered with bristle-like setae. Material fine enough to pass this valve may proceed by a dorsal channel, the mid-gut filter, straight to the mid-gut. Much of it however, seeps downwards between the two heavy side walls, forming the filter press, and after further trituration enters the ventrally placed gland filter. This structure consists of two semicircular plates, concave dorsally and united in the middle line. Attached to the anterior border and free behind like the teeth of an excessively fine comb are a series of chitinous rods, each in turn bearing hair-like setae. Dissolved material that has passed the gland filter is carried into the digestive gland for absorption. The residue is carried up into the press and finally to the mid-gut.

# 5 Filter Feeders

Filter feeding is the straining of fine particles from suspension in water, and is used by most of the sessile marine invertebrates. In one group, the barnacles or Cirripedia, food is collected by a casting net of setal-fringed limbs swept through the water by active muscular work. But in most filter feeders, including the sponges, the polyzoans, the brachiopods, the ascidians, the bivalves and some gastropods and polychaete worms, food gathering proceeds almost wholly by the use of cilia and mucus.

Filter feeding is a continuous process, though achieved with great economy of energy. The suspended food may consist of an almost pure plant diet, as of diatoms and dinoflagellates, though more often of small naked flagellates; or it may include zooplankton and varying elements of organic debris such as dead parts and faeces, and even grains of sand. But whether pure or mingled with material less nutritive, food in suspension is very diffuse, and great volumes of water must be driven through the meshes of the different kinds of filters. The oyster, for example passes thirty times its volume of water through its gills in one hour.

Suspended food, unlike the prey of carnivores, is widespread and automatically obtained. Water currents are set up and drawn from a wide area through filtering screens; the material so concentrated is generally bound into ropes or boluses with mucus – a multitude of small unruly particles would be no sooner collected than dispersed. Current production is the work of powerful flexuous cilia. The particles are sometimes entrapped by stiff, inert comb-like cilia, more often by a lattice-like spread of mucus, and sometimes by both together.

Filtering is generally carried out by specialized structures lying outside the gut, before the mouth is reached, such as the tentacle crown of tube worms, the lophophore of polyzoa and the ctenidia of bivalve molluscs. These need not closely concern us here. However, in one important group of filter feeders, the protochordates, the filtering organs are located within the gut, derived from an enlarged and specialized pharynx that overshadows in complexity all the rest of the digestive tract.

Both the sea-squirts (Ascidiacea) and Amphioxus have a variant of the same type of filtering pharynx (Fig. 5–1). Opening by the mouth in front and leading to the oesophagus behind, this branchial sac is fenestrated with small openings called *stigmata*, perforating the pharynx and the body wall essentially as do the gill slits of a fish. The stigmata are, however, finally subdivided and crossed by horizontal connecting bars to form an open lattice work. The body wall is consequently weakened at this level, and a fold of integument called the atrium encloses the space where the

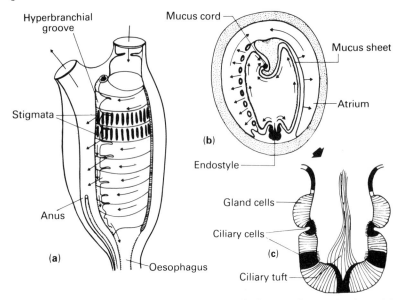

**Fig. 5–1** The structure of the pharynx of the ascidian, *Clavelina*. (a) Diagrammatic vertical section of the pharynx showing the direction of water currents (arrows). (b) Transverse section of the pharynx showing the distribution of mucus. (c) Detailed structure of the endostyle.

slits open. With the atrial cavity laid open, the pharyngeal wall looks somewhat like a limp Aertex singlet. Water drawn in at the mouth is passed through the stigmata to the atrial cavity by current-driving lateral cilia situated along side walls. Particles are strained off and retained within the pharynx by a sheet of mucus that covers the interior surface as a permeable mesh. The mucus is produced by gland cells in the ventral longitudinal groove known as the endostyle; by the action of a median fringe of long cilia at the bottom of the groove, it is wafted outwards in two continuous lateral sheets; other cilia carry it up the sides of the pharynx to the dorsal hyperbranchial groove which runs back to the oesophagus. In many ascidians the movement of mucus is assisted also by the movement of longitudinal folds within the pharynx pushing it like a long broom, with small ciliated papillae acting like brushes. In the hyperbranchial groove a rope of the collected food is fashioned, being held by the ciliated tongues or plain lamina curving round the groove from one side. Backwardly-beating cilia help to carry the food rope to the oesophagus.

The gut behind the pharynx is very simple. The role of the stomach is to receive the food string and make its mucus less viscous by the lowered pH of the medium. As in all ciliary feeders this is the site where the food load is shed, with individual particles set free for digestion and absorption.

The enzymes include protease, amylase and lipase acting extracellularly. They are secreted from special cells in the stomach lining or (in some ascidians) in small diverticula. In the intestine, where the pH rises to more than 7, viscosity of the mucus again increases and a firm string is reconstituted from those particles that are left. By ciliary movements this string is carried repeatedly back and forth across the typhlosole as it passes through the intestine. With fresh accretions of mucus it is fashioned into an elegant faecal rope, firm enough to be discharged from the anus without fouling the ingoing current.

In ascidians the food string is grasped and thrust backwards by oblique ciliated ridges in the oesophagus (Fig. 5–3c). In the lancelet, or Amphioxus, the traction power is exerted from behind by the short section of the intestine known as the ileo-colon ring (Fig. 5–3b). Here strong cilia twist the string into a tight spiral coil and rotate it under moderate tension. The rest of the gut lining is largely set free for other tasks. A dorsal by-pass through the ileo-colon ring allows direct passage to the posterior intestine, while at intervals small pieces of the rotating mucus rope are nipped off and compacted into faeces.

An important feature of the gut of Amphioxus is the digestive diverticulum, running forward from the stomach, alongside the pharynx. The term hepatopancreas should not be applied to this organ: it has none of the functions of the liver which is quite unrepresented in protochordates. A pancreatic role it must, however, be allowed, since it produces a tryptic protease, a lipase and an amylase. The deep-staining, large-nucleated digestive cells are clearly the homologues of those in ascidians, and have been shown to bear a detailed resemblance with the exocrine secreting cells of the pancreas in the higher vertebrate series.

In the pelagic *Salpa* the separate stigmata are replaced by a filtering cone of endostylar mucus, and the pharynx is wide open at either side. Particles are retained as water is pumped, during swimming, through the mucus net, which is wound back into the oesophagus by ciliary rotation. But the most complete and efficient protochordate filterer must be the small appendicularian *Oikopleura*, which uses a pre-oral filter that forms a part of the secreted cuticular 'house' (Fig. 5–2). Long imperfectly understood, its structure has been elucidated by electron microscope studies. The two apparent layers of separate tubes consist of two spaces; the excurrent above, partly divided into tubes by a folded membrane which bounds the continuous incurrent space below. Water is pumped through this system by the oscillation of the 'tail' within the house. The dividing membrane forms a net of fibres, with a mesh of $0.8 \times 0.1 \, \mu$; this is sufficient to hold back the smallest of the nanoplankton. This component of the plankton was first recognized by its discovery in the pre-oral filter of *Oikopleura*.

The Polyzoa are ciliary feeders that use a rotating rod of mucus or faeces to manipulate food particles. The tiny gut of a polyzoan zooid (Fig. 5–3a) forms an exquisite mechanism that can sometimes be seen by

38

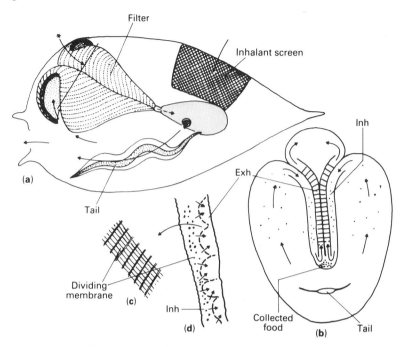

**Fig. 5–2** The filtering system of the appendicularian protochordate, *Oikopleura*. (a) *Oikopleura* in its 'house'; the arrows show the feeding currents. (b) Diagrammatic section taken at the level * (inh – incurrent, exh – excurrent). (c) and (d) Details of the structure of the filtering mechanism.

transparency in the intact animal. Food entering the stomach in the mucus string is engaged by a small swivelling rod, projecting from a thimble-like pylorus, in which it is continually rotated by cilia, at up to 70 turns a minute. The rod points alternately towards the stomach entry where it engages more mucus string with food, and into the large bulb of the stomach where particles are detached and stirred and brought under the action of enzymes. As well as containing gland cells, the stomach lining is freely absorptive and can even phagocytose large diatoms. At intervals the pylorus opens out flat and sucks back the rotating rod into the intestine. Another is gradually built up to replace it, and the rejected rod is kneaded into a faecal pellet in the intestine. Turned by the lining cilia as on a lathe, the pellets are given a final coat of mucus and forcibly expelled from the anus.

The rotating rod of the gut in ciliary feeders has been called by the author the 'ergatula' from a Greek word meaning a 'little capstan'. Its function is to concentrate the work of transport at some special part of the gut; and it is found at its highest development in the Mollusca in which it has acquired other important roles as well. In the bivalve stomach, and

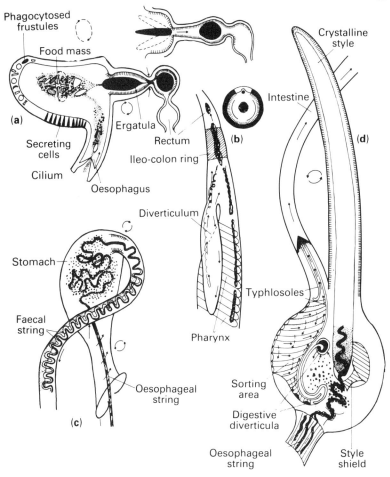

**Fig. 5–3** The guts of some ciliary filter feeders showing the sites of rotation. (**a**) A polyzoan, with (above) changes in the swivelling axis of the ergatula. (**b**) An amphioxus, *Branchiostoma lanceolatum* with a transverse section of the ileo-colon ring. (**c**) The ascidian, *Ciona intestinalis*. (**d**) A bivalve, based on the oyster, *Ostrea edulis*.

among some gastropods, the rotating rod is known as a crystalline style. No longer constructed of faeces, it now forms a column of flexible, hyaline mucoprotein, long, tapering and semitransparent. It projects into the stomach from a special sac, the style caecum, which originated as part of the first section of the intestine, but now in most bivalves lies alongside but completely cut off from the intestine.

The stomach of a bivalve (Fig. 5–3d) is far more complex than that of a polyzoan or protochordate, and to understand its structure it must be remembered that bottom-dwelling bivalves take into the gut a far more mixed flow of debris which requires extensive sorting before final digestion can take place. The winnowing out of the coarse and indigestible from the fine and organic is, of course, more important in those molluscs relying on the surface detrital mantle as their food, less so where the food is a more pure suspension filtered mainly from the water above.

Food is collected by the gill and undergoes preliminary sorting by the labial palps. The mucus strings entering the stomach by the short oesophagus are caught up by the rotating head of the style as it projects from its caecum. The ends of the strings are wound on to the style and rotated with it; they are thrown into a tight coil which in turn draws more material out of the oesophagus. As the string enters, its slack is taken up by progressive winding into the style. Meanwhile the mucus becomes less viscid, owing to the lowered pH of the stomach; food particles are shed and the string itself may be reduced to an axial thread, usually keeping a slender continuity with the style.

The rotating crystalline style is not only a capstan, but also acts as a pestle; it stirs the particles shed from the food string repeatedly over the grooved and ciliated part of the lining of the stomach. This structure forms a ciliary sorting area and separates particles into coarse and lighter fractions. Sorting areas are important in all molluscs, and sometimes they may be extended out of the stomach into a shallow sorting caecum; one such diverticulum is shown in Fig. 5–3d of the oyster's stomach. A typhlosole winds its way into and out of the caecum, and multiple openings of the digestive gland occur there. The coarsest material resulting from sorting is conducted along a ciliated groove, bounded by the typhlosole, directly into the first part of the intestine. The finer particles still remaining undergo some extracellular digestion in the stomach by the action of enzymes coming from two sources: from the detached tips of the cells of the digestive diverticula, and from a powerful amylase liberated from the style as its head becomes softened and dissolved in the weakly acid medium of the stomach. As well as being rotated by powerful cilia, the style is also thrust slowly into the stomach by cilia beating longitudinally towards the opening of the style sac. As it gradually dissolves it is simultaneously renewed by fresh secretion in the caecum, and maintains its constant length as it is pushed downward. Thus, as well as being a capstan and a pestle, the style also serves as an enzyme store – an ideal mechanism for the slow, continuous liberation of small quantities of amylase. The same enzyme comes from the digestive gland, with the addition of protease and lipase.

Particles are absorbed in two ways. The largest digestible material, such as diatoms, may be engulfed by amoebocytic cells that make their way in from the blood spaces beneath the stomach lining. These are especially noteworthy in the oyster where, with the phagocytosed contents, they may retreat into the epithelium or break up to be finally absorbed themselves.

Fine food is ultimately taken up by the cells of the digestive diverticula, and digestion is completed intracellularly (Fig. 1–1b).

The intestine of the bivalve is only moderately long; its role is to divide up the mucus string of waste coming from the stomach and fashion short sections into faecal pellets. These are rounded off and enveloped with clear mucus for final discharge into the mantle cavity.

A number of large vertebrates feed by specialized filtering methods; not that their food is generally of diatoms, but of the much larger zooplankton, including – in the whales – the shrimp-like crustaceans known as euphausiids.

At a smaller level of size, the tadpoles of many frogs and toads are entirely microphagous, while others take the bulk of their food from the water currents passing through their gill filters. Their filtering habit is entirely distinct in its origin from that of protochordates, and the mechanisms are very different in detail. The inhalant current is no longer created by cilia, but the gill pouches develop filters through which water is pumped by muscular action. Most tadpoles still use the jaws for masticatory ingestion, but in the mountain frog, *Ascaphus*, the tadpole's mouth is preoccupied as a holding sucker and the nostrils are used for the feeding and respiratory current. Figure 5–4a shows a longitudinal section

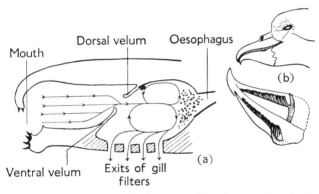

**Fig. 5–4** (a) Diagram of longitudinal section of the pharynx of a tadpole of *Bufo*, showing the movement of water currents and food particles. (After SAVAGE, R. M. (1952). *Proc. zool. Soc. Lond.*, **122**, 467.) (b) Head and upper jaw of the broad-billed prion, *Pachyptila forsteri*, showing the filtering lamellae.

of the mouth and pharynx of a tadpole of *Bufo bufo*. The pharynx is wide and flat so that water is drawn through it as a thin sheet. In front of the gill openings it is partly divided by oblique septa called the dorsal and ventral vela. Water leaving the pharynx passes ventrally through the gill openings which are guarded by lattice-like filters forming a grating that holds back larger particles. Most of the particulate food is, however, thrown towards the oesophagus by centrifugal force, where the water turns through an angle of 180° behind the vela. Mucus is secreted in grooves on either side behind the dorsal velum, and the two food strings so formed are twisted together as they pass down the oesophagus.

Of the marine birds, the leading plankton filterers are the broad-billed prions, *Pachyptila* (Fig. 5–4b). In these the upper part of the bill bears two rows of comb-like lamellae through which skimmed-up plankton is strained; the large fleshy tongue acts as a plunger. Among freshwater birds, the duck tribe have a set of simple bill lamellae or side-strainers. In the flamingoes the gill is developed to a filter of the highest pitch of efficiency. A detailed study of its structure and function, has shown how two African flamingo species can co-exist on the same lakes without competing for food. The small *Phoeniconaias minor* sweeps the bill through the surface water and filters out blue green algae and diatoms. The larger *Phoenicopterus antiquorum* has a coarser filter with which it feeds in the bottom muds on chironomid larvae and other small invertebrates.

Among the pelagic fish, the herring and the mackerel possess long thin gill-rakers which prevent the escape of copepods and other zooplankton. Some of the largest of the sharks, the basking-shark *Cetorhinus* and the whale-shark *Rhinodon*, feed solely on plankton, strained by similar gill rakers. In the whalebone whales, Mystacoceti, the filtering apparatus consists of close-set transverse plates, up to 300 in right whales. As the lower jaw is raised and the tongue is brought close to the roof of the mouth, euphausiid shrimps or 'krill' are strained off by the finely-divided, horny fringes of the baleen plates.

# 6 Fluid Feeders

Almost every kind of plant and animal fluid may be used as food: cell sap or the watery tissues of plants, productions such as nectar or honeydew, the exudates of decay, and the wide variety of liquids and secretions of animals – blood, protein-rich coelomic fluid, egg yolk and albumen, even sweat which is sucked up by butterflies for its salt content. In most of these diets the constituents are pure and fairly easily digestible; the main problems to be surmounted are those of gaining access to fluids in other living organisms, of pumping or sucking them into the gut, and of storing their inevitably large bulk. Where the food is blood, there is the additional problem of preventing coagulation; as well as an anti-coagulant, the saliva sometimes contains an irritant which promotes the supply of blood to the area being sampled.

Some animals that live on body fluids have simplified the whole problem of intake by lying immersed in nutritive fluids and absorbing them straight through the surface of the body. The outer body wall then does duty as a gut, as in the cestode flatworms and in degenerate parasitic barnacles such as *Sacculina*, and even in one endoparasitic gastropod, *Enteroxenos*, living in holothurians.

## 6.1 Insects

Starting with insects that feed on plant fluids, the insect order Hemiptera can be taken as an example. Hemipterans, broadly known as 'bugs', are all suctorial whether on plant or animal food. The piercing stylets are the long flexible mandibles and maxillae; these converge closely as they pass down the groove in the labium. The two maxillae form together a narrower tube for injection of saliva and a wider channel for sucking up food. In a sap feeder such as a coccid, the oesophagus is a simple narrow tube. As in many fluid feeders the mid-gut has lost its peritrophic membrane, protection against hard particles being no longer needed. The stomach is formed by the greatly dilated mid-gut, separated by a sphincter from the long intestine. The most interesting feature of the stomach is the part known as the *filter chamber*. The first and third portions of the mid-gut form extensive coils which lie against each other, enveloped in a fold of the rectum and invisible from the body cavity. The middle part lies free and its histology is very distinct, with vacuolated and secretory cells. Such a topography clearly allows excess fluid to pass from the first to the third part of the mid-gut directly. The middle part, being short-circuited, receives for digestion and absorption only the valuable constituents left after removal of fluid (Fig. 6–1a). Enzyme dilution is also thus avoided. The transfer of fluid is not merely a passive diffusion; the intestinal wall expends energy in active transport. Whether there is a further transit of fluid through the enveloping rectal wall is not known, but this would seem unlikely since the hind part of the mid-gut is directly continuous with the rectum.

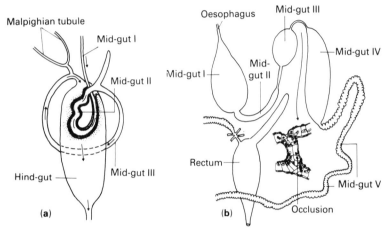

**Fig. 6–1**   Fluid-feeding insects. (a) Gut of the coccid *Lecanium* showing the filtration system between the mid-gut and the hind-gut. (b) Gut of the pentatomid bug *Acanthocoris obscuricornis*, showing details of the occlusion between parts III and IV of the mid-gut.

The fluid excrement of coccids is very copious and contains much unabsorbed organic matter, especially sugars and other carbohydrates, furnishing the familiar honeydew coating the surfaces of leaves. The manna of biblical times seems to have been the honeydew of a coccid, *Trabutina mannipara*, living on tamarisk in Sinai. The vast excess of secreted sugar is surprising (manna contains 55% sucrose, 25% invert sugar  and 19% dextrin). Such large meals of sugary plant juice may perhaps serve to supply the insect's protein needs from the same sources, but this cannot be the whole truth since the excrement may contain up to 5% of unused protein. Some other scarce nutritive substance is probably involved.

The need of accessory factors and trace substances may also explain the occurrence in most plant-sucking Hemiptera of specific microorganisms carefully transmitted from one generation to another. In some insects the bacteria may live in pouches of the mid-gut, but in the coccids they are aggregated in 'mycetomes', strings of modified cells here contained within the fat-body. In blood-sucking insects bacteria occur too, but only in those taking a narrow diet of blood at all stages; sterile mammalian blood is an incomplete food and the bacteria are probably responsible for vitamin production (Fig. 6–2a).

Fig. 6–1b shows the mid-gut of a shield bug, with its four regions: I – a capacious sac, II – a slender tube, III – a smaller sac and IV – a further bulbous portion followed by a narrow tube with small saccules. These insects take highly pure food and discontinuities lie between parts III and IV of the mid-gut and sometimes between parts IV and V. Such occlusions of the gut are also found in larvae of Hymnoptera and Neuroptera that are given food which has been processed by the adult and so contains little, if any, indigestible residue to be passed to the intestine.

The salivary glands and their secretions in the honey bee are complex and diverse (Fig. 6–2a). First there are the mandibular glands producing

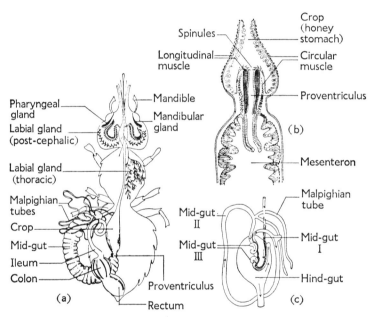

**Fig. 6–2**    (a) Alimentary canal of the honey bee, *Apis mellifica*. (b) Longitudinal section of the crop or honey stomach, proventriculus and mesenteron.

an acid secretion (pH 4.6–4.8); they are very active in the queen, less so in the workers and vestigial in the drones. Their secretion perhaps assists the softening of the cocoon at emergence. The second pair of glands, the pharyngeal glands, produce during the early life of the adult the royal jelly used in feeding the young stages of the queens. The bee requires pollen for these glands to become fully active, which happens 3–6 days after emergence. (The secretion has an acid reaction of pH 4.5–5.0.) When foraging begins at three weeks the glands switch over to the secretion of amylase and invertase, becoming most active at about a month, and being responsible for the presence of these enzymes in honey. The appearance of invertase at the onset of foraging is a good example of the phased production of enzymes in response to current metabolic needs. The third salivary glands, the labial glands, are in two divisions: posterior cephalic with a natural secretion of a fatty emulsion to work wax, and thoracic glands active throughout life, and producing no enzyme but a watery secretion (pH 6.3–7.0) probably used in comb-building.

Among the social Hymenoptera, the bees have developed a perfect apparatus for taking nectar which is converted to honey in the dilated crop known as the 'honey stomach' (Fig. 6–2b). No absorption takes place here and the exit to the mid-gut is guarded by the honey stopper, a special projection from the proventriculus. The lumen of the honey stopper is occluded by four converging, spinose lips. Pollen grains are seized by these and transferred without crushing into the mid-gut, leaving behind the fluid nectar. In a bee fed on a suspension of syrup with pollen grains the crop will remain tense with fluid while pollen is gradually removed. The grains are then separately digested, probably by enzymes reaching the pollen starch through the open micropyle. The waste from a meal is relatively small and may be long retained; in the young imago the hugely distended rectum is not evacuated until foraging begins three weeks after hatching.

A number of insects are specialized for drawing off blood from living animals. The most important are the blood-sucking Hemiptera (such as *Cimex* and *Rhodnius*), the fleas (Siphonaptera) and the blood-sucking true flies or Diptera, including gnats, mosquitoes and the tsetse flies, *Glossina*. The last-named shows us a good example of the gut of a fluid-feeding dipteran (Fig. 6–3). The lancing and sucking mouth parts lack the stylets formed by the mandibles and maxillae in the mosquito; the labium forms a sharp chitinized probe and along it runs an injection needle, the hypopharynx, and a suction tube, the epipharynx. The saliva driven down the hypopharynx is not enzymic but contains an irritant and also keeps the mouth parts clean between feeding. It also provides in *Glossina* a powerful anticoagulin. If the salivary glands are removed the proboscis and crop become blocked with blood clots, but until this occurs feeding proceeds normally.

Blood passes straight to the crop, which in most Diptera is a diverticulum opening by a narrow duct and storing great amounts of fluid, to be released and passed on in small instalments. In those mosquitoes that take sugary plant juices as well, these alone are stored in the crop, the blood meal being carried straight to the stomach.

The mid-gut of *Glossina* shows great histological variation and division of labour. In the anterior segment the lining cells are pale-staining; the blood here becomes friable by the absorption of water, but no digestion occurs. Over a short length there is a zone of cells containing rod-like symbiotic bacteria. In the middle segment the cells are large and deep staining, secreting enzymes, and the blood becomes blackened in contact with this epithelium. Carbohydrases are very feeble, but the proteases are

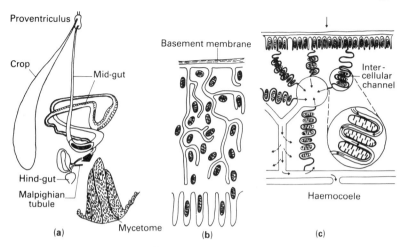

**Fig. 6–3** (a) Gut of the tsetse fly, *Glossina* with detail of the mycetomal region of the mid-gut. (b) Detailed structure of the epithelium of the Malpighian tubule. (c) Diagrammatic representation of the structure of the rectal papillae and the pathway of water absorption. The drawing is based on *Periplaneta* (see Fig. 2–5), but the general scheme would apply to dipterans. (After MADDRELL, S. (1971). *Adv. Insect Physiol.*, 8, 199.)

highly active, being secreted under the stimulus of feeding; the medium is slightly acid (pH 6.5–6.6). The third segment, the narrow posterior part of the stomach, is lined with absorptive cells.

The Malpighian tubules and the rectal glands are the water-regulating organs associated with the insect gut. The Malpighian tubules have a strongly folded basal border, with indentations reaching almost to the apical border, and numerous mitochondria (Fig. 6–3b). The rectal glands in dipterans form large papillae projecting into the gut lumen. The apical cell membrane is folded into regular leaflets which, together with the regular stacks of membrane-lined channels formed from the lateral cell borders and folded into intercellular spaces, are closely associated with mitochondria. Water and ions pass along these intercellular spaces from the rectum to the haemolymph, but apically and basally the cells are tight sealed by septate desmosomes (Fig. 6–3c).

## 6.2   Suctorial molluscs

The opisthobranchs have become diversely specialized for suctorial feeding and most of them are carnivorous on sessile or encrusting animals (Fig. 6–4). The dorid opisthobranchs originated as rasping feeders on sponges, with a typical odontophore and radula. The slugs of the genus *Dendrodoris* have wholly lost the radula, and a prolonged muscular proboscis penetrates a sponge body or ascidian test by an

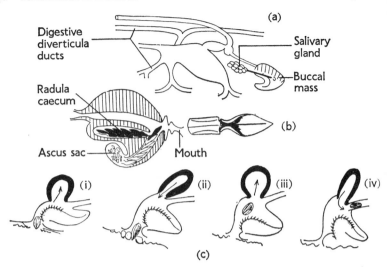

**Fig. 6–4** Suctorial opisthobranchs. (a) Diagram of the gut of *Alderia modesta*. (After EVANS, T. J. (1952). *Proc. malacol. Soc. London.*, **29**, 249.) (b) Sagittal section of the buccal mass of *Alderia* with a single, much enlarged tooth. (c) *Okenia plana* – stages in the action of the radula and buccal pump in removing a zooid from the polyzoan *Zoobotryon*.

enzymic salivary secretion. *Onchidoris* and *Okenia* suck out the whole zooids of polyzoan colonies, using a bulb-shaped pharyngeal pump. The mouth fastens to the top of a zooecium, the radula works with rapid strokes, and the buccal pump dilates to provide a suction force that draws the contents out of the horny zooecial wall. With the zooid removed, the mouth closes, and the pumping of the bulb now forces it along the oesophagus (Fig. 6–4c).

The aeoliid nudibranchs are carnivorous upon coelenterates, and have evolved a relationship with the stinging cells, or nematocysts, of their prey. These remain unexploded when the food is eaten, and become arranged in the epithelium of the cnidosac, a small chamber opening at the tip of each of the cerata and inwardly continuous with the digestive diverticulum. From here, the nematocysts can be shot out to the exterior when the aeoliid is irritated or attacked (Fig. 6–5a).

*Calma glaucoides* (Fig. 6–5b), a modified aeoliid slug that crawls over egg clusters of blennioid fish, and fits over the egg a 'face' like a hood, has a special suctorial habit. The egg is too large and slippery to be swallowed, neither can it be chewed lest its fluid contents be washed away. It is thus firmly held by the folds of the lips and incised with three sharp processes, the edges of the jaws and the median radula. Yolk produces few or no faeces, and the anus is closed, wastes accumulating in the digestive gland through life.

Very different from nudibranch slugs are the minute, long-spired

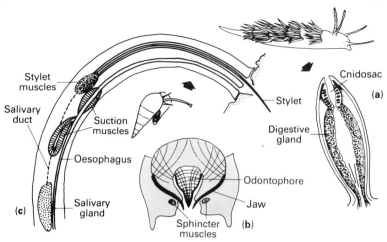

**Fig. 6–5**   Suctorial molluscs. (a) Single ceras of an aeoliid nudibranch showing the open terminal cnidosac. (b) Vertical section of the mouth and buccal mass of *Calma glaucoides*. (c) *Odostomia*, a pyramidellid snail, with the proboscis shown in longitudinal section.

snails that live ectoparasitically on the bodies of bivalves, tubeworms and coelenterates. In the Pyramidellidae (*Odostomia, Turbonilla, Chrysallida*), the thread-like proboscis contains a slender stylet, formed by the attenuation of the fused jaws, and perforated by a salivary duct (Fig. 6–5c). This is used for piercing the integument to take blood or body fluids. The pharynx muscles form a sucking pump, and the ampullae of the salivary glands also have pumping muscles. No trace of the radula remains. In the convergently evolved Eulimidae (*Balcis*) living with echinoderms, there are neither hard parts nor salivary glands, and the eversible proboscis is inserted into host tissues evidently softened by the secretion of enlarged pedal glands of the attaching foot.

An important section of the opisthobranchs, the small greenish and black slugs of the order Sacoglossa, are suctorial herbivores, specialized for feeding on the cell contents of green algae. The radula is peculiarly fashioned, lying in a >-shaped tube, opening at its angle through the floor of the pharynx. Only one tooth is in use at a time, and these originate in the upper limb of the tube, and worn teeth detaching and passing into the lower limb. Sacoglossans are highly specific in their food plants, and the teeth, which form tiny pointed blades, are beautifully adapted to the cell size of the species concerned. Thus the British *Alderia modesta* sucks out the cell contents of *Vaucheria* with a filament diameter of $40–60\,\mu$ and its dental cusp is $33–35\,\mu$ long. The mode of feeding is very elegant: a kink of the filament is drawn between the lips of the mollusc and the cells lanced rapidly with a lengthwise incision; the colourless end of the filament is passed out, with its cells slit open and emptied of green contents. The radula cusp is both a scalpel and a spoon, and as many as ten cells can be dealt with in a minute. The pharynx forms a powerful force pump, its roof being highly contractile, working in concert with an oesophageal valve near the entrance to the stomach. The stomach is merely a small annexe to the intestine, and provides openings to the long-branched digestive diverticula which enter the club-shaped outgrowths of the back, or cerata. The fluid gut contents flow freely in these, and impart their general colour to the animal. The chloroplasts of the alga are aggregated into spherules in the gut and can be seen to stream in and out of the diverticula by regular pulsations of the cerata. Recent research has made it clear that intact chloroplasts can remain photosynthetic, and enter into a symbiotic relation with a slug.

## 6.3   Arachnida

All these arthropods, including spiders, scorpions, ticks and mites, are essentially suctorial feeders, even when they prey upon the whole bodies of larger animals. The spiders (Fig. 6–6a) inject a strong salivary protease into the body of the prey, together with a disabling toxin contributed from the cheliceral glands. A captured fly is held close to the mouth by the pedipalps and the saliva is extruded drop by drop until the proteins are liquefied and digested, leaving the skin an empty husk within a few hours. The narrow pharynx acts as a muscular pump to draw this fluid into the gut. The rest of the digestive tract provides all the room possible for great periodic intake of fluid. First, in the 'thorax' or prosoma, there are two large lateral caeca branching into the legs. Further back, in the 'abdomen' or opisthosoma, the diverticula are much finer and massed together in a soft, brownish grey, semifluid digestive gland. All this spacious system appears to be both absorptive and digestive: the gland cells secrete further enzymes into the ingested broth and other cells – or the same cells in a different phase – ingest and absorb. Senescent cells break up and form granules of faecal matter, which is sparse and voided only at long intervals; together with excretions from the Malpighian tubules, it accumulates in a plump stercoral pocket in the wall of the rectum.

The blood-sucking mites and ticks (Acarina) have similar ingestive arrangements, further specialized. The salivary duct runs forward to bring a supply of anticoagulin to the incision site. Blood is forced through the sucking pharynx into a capillary oesophagus which opens into the stomach. This is the meeting place for several pairs of caeca, very spacious, especially the lateral pair. Completely collapsible when empty, they become tensely inflated after a meal, the oesophageal valve preventing regurgitation from the stomach. As the stomach is distended, its lining cells stretch to a thin pavement and long glandular cells stretch far out into the lumen. These increase the digestive surface by penetrating into the blood mass, phagocytosing part-digested food. Their tips may be nipped off to liberate enzymes, and the effete cells yield up blackish

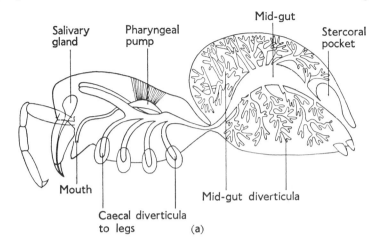

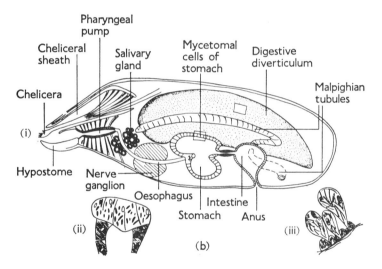

**Fig. 6–6** (a) Gut of a spider, showing the arrangement of the diverticula. (b) Gut of the bird mite, *Ornithonyssus bacoti*: (i) whole animal in sagittal section; (ii) details of mycetomal cells; (iii) detail of pseudopodial digestive cells.

granules of excrement. In the tick, *Ixodes*, the stomach may be cut off from the intestine and excrement is stored during the life in distended pseudopodial cells, leaving the intestine simply as a conduit from the Malpighian tubules.

As in blood-sucking insects, the stomach wall of mites and ticks carries a patch of large cells containing microorganisms and forming a mycetome. With a special diet of restricted content, the farming of these symbionts probably secures a supply of vitamins or other essential traces lacking from the food (Fig. 6–6b).

## 6.4   Leeches

The Hirudinea form a whole class of annelid worms given over to ectoparasitic blood sucking. The small freshwater *Glossiphonia*, feeding from molluscs such as *Lymnea* and *Planorbis*, gives a representative picture of the parts of a leech's gut (Fig. 6–7). The muscular proboscis receives at

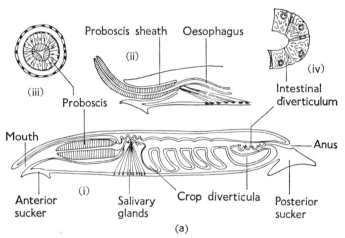

**Fig. 6–7**   Gut of the freshwater leech, *Glossiphonia*: (i) whole animal in section, (ii) proboscis extended, with (iii) detail of proboscis in transverse section, and (iv) cells of intestinal diverticulum, containing symbionts.

its base the ducts of numerous salivary glands. A narrow oesophagus leads back to a stomach with five pairs of spacious lateral caeca. The short intestine has four pairs of tiny diverticula, the lining of which forms a mycetome with symbiotic bacteria.

The course of digestion has been studied most in the medicinal leech *Hirudo*, which differs from *Glossiphonia* in having no proboscis but an armature of sharp jaws. The saliva contains a powerful anticoagulin. Massive blood meals are stored in the caeca of the stomach which become distended to as much as ten times the leech's normal volume at a single meal. For days the blood undergoes no noticeable change – even its precipitins, antibodies and pathogenic bacteria can still be detected amidst a deposit of haemoglobin crystals. After weeks or months a process of haemolysis can be observed; in the epithelial lining cells, haemoglobin is broken down to haem and globin. The latter is used in metabolism and biosynthesis, the haem being transformed to colouring matter and its iron largely excreted. The enzymes of *Hirudo* have been little studied; they include a powerful protease, but lipase is apparently absent.

# 7 Return to Photosynthesis

One of the first stages in animal evolution was the loss of the autotrophic system of nutrition; it is almost a definition of animals that they cannot photosynthesize. However, many animals, particularly filterers and other microphages, have adopted a symbiotic relationship with unicellular algae. Zoochlorellae and zooxanthellae, as they are called, are found captive in the tissues of many invertebrates. The green hydra, *Chlorohydra viridissima*, has, for example, *Chlorella* cells in a balanced symbiosis in the gastrodermis cells of the coelenteron. The acoelan flatworm *Convoluta roscoffensis* abandons food ingestion early in life and then lives on the huge numbers of algae, a chlamydomonad, *Carteria*, present in the mesenchyme. When these are exhausted it dies after laying eggs supplied with an infective 'seeding' of algae for the new generation.

The hermatypic reef corals, living in warm, shallow and well-lighted waters, characteristically harbour zooxanthellae (the vegetative form of the mobile dinoflagellate *Gymnodinium*) within the gastrodermis. Reef corals are efficient microcarnivores and are not dependent on their algae for nutrition, Coral nutrition is not impaired in the dark, though the zooxanthellae are extruded in sustained absence of light and passed into the gut through the mesenterial filaments.

One of the advantages gained by the imprisoned phytoplankton is metabolic access to the phosphate, $CO_2$, ammonia, guanine, adenine and uric acid produced by the host.

The belief that algae account for the high primary production of reefs has been shown to be false, but the symbionts do assist calcium deposition in the corals. Calcium deposition is markedly reduced in the dark (in *Manicina* falling to 50% on a rainy day). Figure 7–1a shows the pathways of calcium and carbonate metabolism. Calcium is taken up from sea-water through the cells lining the coelenteron, and after active transport is absorbed on a mucopolysaccharide organic matrix and incorporated as bicarbonate. $H_2CO_3$ is then removed, leaving $CaCO_3$ for skeletal deposition. Carbonic anhydrase breaks down $H_2CO_3$ to $CO_2$ and water, and zooxanthellae metabolizes the $CO_2$.

Although the stony corals derive no food from their zooxanthellae, some of the Alcyonacea have evolved a much closer dependence on a photosynthetic food source. The best known are the individual or colonial polyps, *Xenia*. These have mesenteries crowded with zooxanthellae, and die when they are extruded in the dark; the mouth is used only for ciliary-driven respiratory currents. Certain of the tropical *Alcyonium* species, and the soft corals, *Lobophytum* and *Sarcophyton*, form a series with increasing algal dependence.

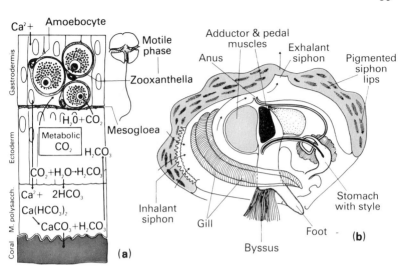

**Fig. 7–1** Symbiotic zooxanthellae. (a) Diagram of a section of the body of a polyp showing the suggested pathways of secretion of the coral skeleton. (Based on GOREAU, T. F. (1956). *Biol. Bull.*, **116**, 59.) (b) Schematic vertical section of the giant clam, *Tridacna*. (After YONGE, C. M. (1953). *Proc. zool. Soc. Lond.*, **123**, 551.)

The largest of the bivalve molluscs, the giant clams, also maintain farms of zooxanthellae exposed to the light in sun-warmed shallow waters. The giant clam (Fig. 7–1b) is oriented so that the toothed gap faces upwards, to display the greatly expanded siphonal lips which are strikingly pigmented in shades of green, blue, brown and yellow. Zooxanthellae (now known to be the immotile stage of the free flagellate *Gymnodinium micro-adriaticum*) live in immense numbers in these illuminated tissues; enclosed in the clam's own amoebocytes they migrate abundantly into the visceral mass, but do not occur in the gut cells. Unlike the reef corals, it seems clear that the clams derive from the algae an important addition to their nutrient supply. They far exceed any other bivalves in size, though the plankton-filtering ctenidia, the stomach and crystalline style are relatively small. Isotope-labelling experiments have shown that the nutrients obtained by the clam derive from photosynthesis and not the digestion of zooxanthellae.

These findings on clams have been paralleled by studies on the symbiotic chloroplasts taken from cell sap of green algae by the sacoglossan slug *Tridachia*. The nutrient benefit is again from the products of photosynthesis.

# 8 Practical Work

The first and most engrossing laboratory work on the gut will be found in the study of its adaptive design. As the previous pages should have made clear, structure and function must be considered together – and more than any other of the major systems the gut lends itself to observation as a working system.

Useful laboratory material will be found in the various invertebrates in which the processes of the living gut can be watched in the intact animal. Best of all are probably the Crustacea. *Daphnia*, the water-flea, displays the full gut by transparency when immobilized in a cavity slide and its movements can be seen clearly. With slightly more difficulty the workings of the gastric mill of a prawn can be seen through the transparent carapace of the animal viewed under a binocular microscope. A cockroach with the wings removed and imprisoned in a wax chamber between two glass slides will – with sufficient transmitted light – show the movements of the various parts of the gut, particularly the action of the teeth in the proventriculus. The same observations can be made after removal of the dorsal body wall and placing the roach in insect perfusion fluid. Small transparent leeches such as *Glossiphonia* also make good material for the study of the live gut.

For observation of the rotating protostyle within the stomach there are two excellent sources of material. Living polyzoans, such as *Bugula* and *Membranipora*, can be viewed intact with the low power of the microscope showing the spinning of the pyloric rod, the movements of the stomach and the formation of faeces. Oyster spat, another good subject, should be collected fresh at the eyespot stage from between the gill lamellae of the parent *Ostrea edulis*. The rotations of the crystalline style can be readily observed and counted, as also the rhythmic contractile movements pumping material to and from the digestive diverticula. Feeding the spat with small green flagellates will allow observation of the course of digestion in the diverticula.

The use of indicators on the living gut demonstrates its range in pH values, with changes appropriate to control mucus viscosity or enzyme activity. Neutral red is a suitable wide range indicator which in dilute (0.02%) solution can be employed to stain whole animals such as *Daphnia* or oyster spat. Below pH 6 it is red; rose at pH 7, orange at pH 8, yellow at pH 9. Better sensitivity may be obtained with several of the BDH indicators selected to cover different parts of the range. With larger animals gut fluids can be mixed with indicator for colour comparison in capillator tubes.

Methods for enzyme study can be applied to a wide variety of guts that can be assayed for digestive activity. Active extracts from small animals can be prepared by grinding pieces of gut in a little mortar made by roughening the bottom of a glass concavity with carborundum. Rinse with distilled water, making up to appropriate dilution and centrifuge. Add 1 ml of the clear supernatant to the same amount of the substrate in a small test-tube and incubate at say, 25°C, for an hour or longer.

For amylase tests use a 1% starch solution, measuring the progress of digestion by mixing a drop of substrate with a drop of iodine on a porcelain plate. Loss of blue colour indicates completion of digestion; or the whole sample can be made blue with iodine and the time of reaching end-point noted. Test on completion with Fehling's or Benedict's solution for the production of reducing sugar. Solutions of the crystalline style of molluscs should be tested for amylolytic action.

For invertase use a sucrose substrate, testing with Fehling's or Benedict's solution (for details see any elementary physiology manual). A good substrate for cellulase detection can be made by digesting high quality filter papers with concentrated sulphuric acid, repeatedly washing the white pulp so produced and making a pale suspension in distilled water of a little of the powdery precipitate. The course of digestion, with the removal of fine cellulose particles from the suspension, can be followed by measuring the decreasing optical density of the suspension with a photoelectric absorptiometer. Test finally or at known intervals with Fehling's or Benedict's solution for the production of reducing sugars.

Protein digestion can be studied most simply by incubating drops of the suspected gut extract upon the gelatin film of a developed photographic plate and noting after a given time the amount of erosion. Flakes of Congo-red-stained fibrin can be observed at intervals with the microscope. A better quantitative method, however, is to note the progressive digestion of small cubes of hard-boiled egg white, or of egg white in specially prepared 'Mett' tubes. These are made by filling 15 cm lengths of 1–2 mm glass tubing with strained egg albumen, sealing both ends in a flame and coagulating in boiling water. Cut into 1.5 cm lengths for use and record extent and rate of dissolution of the albumen column. Amino acid production may be tested for at end-point or at intervals by the standard procedure of formal titration.

Enzyme studies of the gut can be systematically carried out, region by region, and a chart drawn up showing the various enzymes present and their sites of greatest activity. The efficiency of the fluid gut contents should also be compared with that of contact digestion by the epithelial wall. Good results are obtained in this way with the mesenteric filaments of anemones. Cubes of liver or egg white may be offered to an intact anemone, and after a time interval extracted from the coelenteron to show their close investment by a coating of mesenteric filaments.

Experiments to ascertain the activity of enzymes with variation of temperature and of pH can easily be set up with the use of a simple waterbath or with pH controlled buffered solutions.

The saliva of medicinal leeches or of the land-leech, *Haemopus*, may be tested for the presence of an anticoagulin. Add a drop of salivary gland extract to a 1 ml sample of mammalian blood. Using as a control an extract of any other convenient invertebrate tissue, compare the times for coagulation in the two preparations. The thorax of a mosquito may be dissected for the salivary glands, or crushed and extracted, and a micro-test for anticoagulin can be devised on similar lines. The mouth parts of the mosquito or of the bed-bug, *Cimex*, may be watched in action on the bare skin, and the inflation with blood of the crop diverticulum seen through the body wall. With the medicinal leech note the painless incision, the withdrawal of blood, and the triangular mark left by the jaws, as well as the continued flow of blood. Afterwards cleanse the site of incision carefully with antiseptic.

Histological preparations should be studied as widely as opportunity offers. The extent and thickness of the muscular wall should be noted in relation to the strength of peristalsis. The location and appearance of different types of epithelial cells, such as mucus-producing, ciliary and absorbing, may also be studied. In filter-feeding animals, the distribution of mucus can be beautifully revealed by several histological methods. Sections should be lightly stained in eosin, followed by the metachromatic stain thionine, giving various shades of mauve, purple, and black. Alternatively, after light haematoxylin or haemalum staining, mucus can be detected by its deep red reaction with mucicarmine.

Sites of absorption can be detected by the Prussian blue method, after feeding with materials containing powdered iron saccharate or other suitable iron compounds. Particles taken up by the cells can be demonstrated *in situ* by placing the sections, before staining, in potassium ferrocyanide to obtain a deep blue precipitate. Absorption of particles by amoebocytes can be well studied in sections from the stomach of suitably fed sea-urchins. Stomach contents can be carefully withdrawn from living mussels or oysters by inserting a cannula along the oesophagus at intervals after feeding. A useful experimental diet is that of nucleated red blood corpuscles of a fish in faint pink suspension in sea-water. Various stages of digestion of the haemoglobin and the nucleus can then be identified. In the oyster it should be possible to see the fed corpuscles engulfed by the bivalve's own amoebocytes, or lodged in the lining epithelial cells. Van Gieson's picrofuchsin is a useful stain to identify haemoglobin, in fixed sections, by the distinctive greenish colour imparted. In stomach contents of bivalves, spherules and waste droplets from the digestive gland can be identified in their various stages. Large and inert particles, easily identifiable, such as the diatom frustules in Kieselguhr (diatomaceous earth) may be administered to living bivalves; their distribution in sections reveals the areas of sorting and waste disposal.

Ciliary action can sometimes be watched in intact transparent guts. In larger animals the workings of the ciliary systems can be seen by carefully opening the living stomach and viewing with the binocular microscope under sea-water or perfusion fluid. Bivalves such as mussels or oysters are most likely to give good results. Small amounts of carmine-stained starch or carborundum powder may be pipetted on to the ciliated surfaces. The course of ciliary currents can sometimes be deduced from the fixed stomach by the shape and twisting of mucus strings, the location of rejected waste and the composition of faeces.

The most straightforward study of ciliary action can be made in the food-collecting ctenidia of a bivalve such as the sea-mussel, *Mytilus*. Ciliary sorting can also be observed on the inner faces of the labial palps of bivalves, where it closely resembles the same process in the interior of the stomach. The heaviest particles are rejected along grooves, the lightest kept afloat and eventually carried to the mouth. A preparation of the palp, carefully pinned out under sea-water can be presented with a mixture of recognizable particles of different sizes and weights, such as carmine, carborundum, diatomaceous earth, etc. Examining with the binocular, one can note the differences in the way such particles are disposed of; or, after allowing a bivalve to feed on such a mixture, differences may be looked for in the original composition and in that of the material pipetted from the stomach.

The symbiotic microorganisms of various guts can often be clearly seen. Especially good collections of living flagellates are made by washing out with distilled water the rectum of termites and cellulose-feeding cockroaches. From the ruminant stomach, the ciliate protozoa need more careful precautions for study. If the laboratory is close to an abbatoir, or better still to a research station dealing with mammalian physiology, a vacuum flask of fresh rumen contents may be obtained, kept at blood temperature from the outset. Drops of this material, a greenish soup permeated with grass fragments, will show active *Entodinium* and other ciliates, but even a few minutes' drop in temperature will immobilize and kill them.

Whatever the variety of living material, the study of form and adaptation is still likely to be based in large part on the dissecting of preserved animals, the oldest and still the most instructive resource of the morphologist. Well-fixed material is always the most satisfactory to dissect first and generally gives the clearest morphological picture to the beginner. Thereafter all the various methods and techniques can be employed to examine the gut alive. Never neglect in dissecting to open the gut and view its interior thoroughly; the most valuable information lies within. Do not undervalue simple, straightforward methods of quick investigation: razorcut whole sections of the whole fixed animal or its gut are among the most useful of all.

Fixation with Bouin's fluid is recommended for general purposes, followed by several days' washing and hardening in 80% alcohol.

# Further Reading

ANNISON, E. F. and LEWIS, D. (1959). *Metabolism in the Rumen*. Methuen, London.

BARRINGTON, E. J. W. (1941). *Phil. Trans. Roy. Soc. B.*, **228**, 269. (Amphioxus)

BARRINGTON, E. J. W. (1962). Digestive Enzymes I. *Adv. Comp. Physiol. Biochem.*, **1**, 1–65.

*BELL, G. H., EMSLIE-SMITH, D., and PATERSON, C. R. (1976). *Textbook of Physiology and Biochemistry*, 9th edn. E. & S. Livingstone, Edinburgh. (Man)

BIDDER, A. M.(1950). *Quart. J. Micr. Sci.*, **91**, 1. (Cephalopoda)

FARNER, D. S. (1960). Chapter 11 in *Biology and Comparative Physiology of Birds*, vols. 1 and 2. Edited by A. J. MARSHALL. Academic Press, New York and London. (Birds)

*FRETTER, V. and GRAHAM, A. (1962). *British Prosobranch Molluscs*. Ray Society, London. (Gastropoda)

GRAHAM, A.(1949). *Trans. Roy. Soc. Edin.*, **61**, 737. (Molluscan stomach)

GRASSE, P. P., Ed. (1959). Annélides, in *Traité de Zoologie*, tome 5, fasc. 1. Masson et Cie., Paris. (Leech)

HOWELLS, H. H.(1942). *Quart. J. Micr. Sci.*, **83**, 357. (*Aplysia*)

HUGHES, T. E.(1959). *Mites, or the Acari*. Athlone Press, London. (Mites)

KERMACK, D. M.(1955). *Proc. Zool. Soc. Lond.*, **125**, 347. (*Arenicola*)

MILLAR, R. H. (1953). *Ciona*. L.M.B.C. Memoir 25. Liverpool Univ. Press, Liverpool. (Ascidians)

*MORTON, J. E.(1960). *Biol. Rev.*, **35**, 92–140. (Ciliary feeders)

NICOL, J. A. C.(1959). *J. Mar. Biol. Ass. U.K.*, **38**, 469. (Anemone)

STOTT, F. C.(1955). *Proc. Zool. Soc. Lond.*, **125**, 63. (*Echinus*)

*WIGGLESWORTH, V. B. (1972). *Principles of Insect Physiology*, 7th edn. Chapman and Hall, London.

YONGE, C. M.(1924). *J. Exp. Biol.*, **1**, 343. (*Nephrops*)

YONGE, C. M.(1926). *J. Mar. Biol. Ass. U.K.*, **14**, 295. (*Ostrea*)

YONGE, C. M.(1937). *Biol. Rev.*, **12**, 87. (Metazoan digestive system)

* These works contain particularly useful bibliographies.